Smart Muscles Smart Brain

Learn the **somatic movement** way to retrain tight muscles, reduce pain, improve posture and move well through life

Emily Harrison

Smart Muscles Smart Brain
Learn the somatic movement way to retrain tight muscles, reduce pain, improve posture and move well through life

Cover design by Adele Del Signore

ISBN: 978-0-6486434-0-1 (paperback)

A catalogue record for this book is available from the National Library of Australia.

Other formats:

978-0-6486434-1-8 (ebook)
978-0-6486434-2-5 (audio)

Published by Emagination Print.

Medical disclaimer: The information contained in this book is for educational purposes only. It is not intended as medical advice or as a substitute for clinical care. The content is informational and is not designed to diagnose, treat, cure or prevent any condition or disease.

Always consult a healthcare provider for guidance specific to you and before beginning any new movement practice. Explore the physical movements only if you have been cleared to do so. The movement exercises in this book are undertaken at one's own risk.

The author and publisher does not accept any responsibility for issues or circumstances arising from the use of information or instruction contained in this book.

To being, human.
And the human body, my greatest teacher.

Contents

Introduction

My story

I will never quite know if I found somatic movement or if it found me.

We met at a time and place when movement had become painful.

I had started to associate movement with pain. I had even begun to fear it and whether it would mean several days of crippling soreness, restriction and fatigue to come.

The irony was not lost on me, that I, a trained yoga teacher, thought I understood movement. But I was being humbled, schooled from within.

As humans we're wired to move away from pain and discomfort, an inbuilt evolutionary survival mechanism. But what happens when the pain moves with us...or is in us?

The low point came, when sitting across from yet another specialist, they were telling me just how important movement was, and perhaps I should try, yoga.

Intellectually, I also knew this – movement *is* important. Movement is life. But in reality, in my reality, I was having a very different physical experience.

To the outside would, you couldn't tell. I was relatively young, and looked well. Inside felt like a very different story.

And so naturally, I catastrophised...

If I hurt this much, this young, then what sort of future would there be?

Was it always going to be like this? Because this didn't feel like living any sort of life, this felt like being on the sidelines, watching it go by, and wondering why.

And then what if it gets worse...

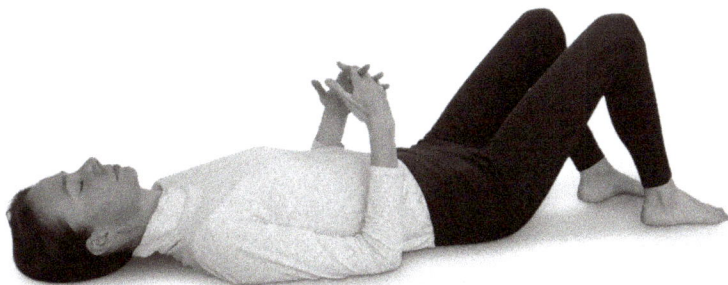

But just as debilitating as pain can be, it can also be an incredible motivator.

And when you've exhausted the conventional then you become pretty open to different possibilities.

So when I stumbled into this 'somatic thing' it was never with the view to becoming a practitioner or eventually writing a book – this book. It was, at the beginning, just a short setup movement practice. It was a way in, a means so that I could continue with yoga, or then the rest of my day, and have less pain.

I noticed that if I did some of these slow gentle floor-based movements, then I wouldn't have the same level of pain, muscle-ache, fatigue or debilitation afterwards or in the days to come.

What happened was my curiosity.

The time I spent rolling on the floor, exploring these movements, became longer and longer. So much so that it felt enough. Like a complete practice. I felt good. I didn't need or want to add something else.

I appeared to have found something quite profound.

I wanted to learn more. I wanted to understand. I am someone that likes to know a clear 'why' behind things.

Yet when I looked around, there were no somatic movement teachers near me and no clinical practitioners even in my country. This was a time well before online classes or courses.

It seemed I needed a me to work with. So I became the teacher that I had needed, embarking on the long path of formal trainings and certifications.

First it was for myself. To understand and embody this, from the inside out. Then it became about sharing it with others.

These movements had felt like such an empowering tool and that they should be shared if someone wanted or was willing to learn. If it resonated for them, in the same way that it had for me.

Because when I first began, I had spent so much time rolling about on the floor, not really knowing why or what I was doing.

I recognised that my long scenic rolling journey could have been a lot quicker, efficient and effective. Not only would that have saved me time, it would have helped me out of pain, discomfort and restriction much sooner.

So often in life there is a long way and a direct way.

Now, when I get to consider how I teach and offer this to clients, then this is the guide, the resource that I wished I had to begin with.

I took the long the road so others don't have to.

In the years since, the online world has dramatically changed and we can now access amazing movement resources from all over the world. In fact, it has almost gone the opposite way and there is so much information and options available.

Amidst this noise and the promise of quick fixes, I have still found these foundational somatic movements to be the slow answer to fast relief and empowering change.

The exercises give us a movement toolkit – something we can learn, use and take with us throughout life. So that we can participate in life!

This is the smart muscles, smart brain way.

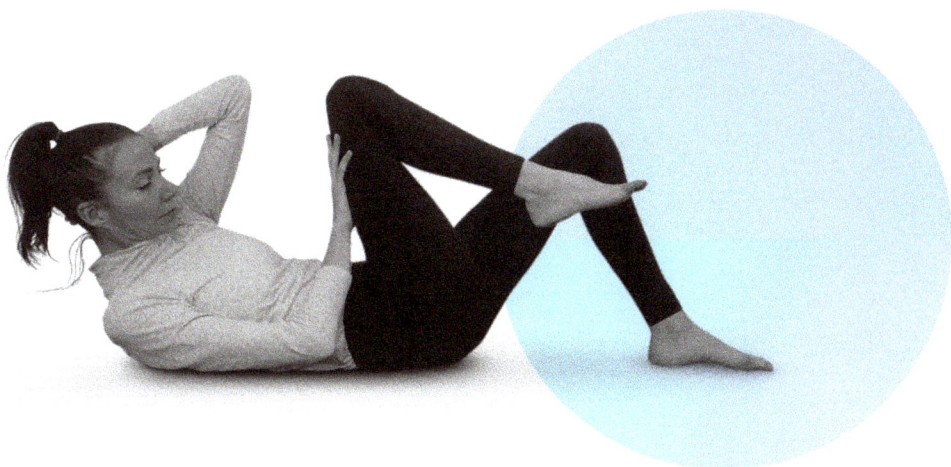

What is somatics?

'What is this somatic thing?' is a question I get asked quite a lot.

The word itself, somatics, comes from the origin of the Greek word 'soma,' meaning of the body or pertaining to the body.

As such, in something 'somatic,' there's going to be an emphasis on the internal, the physical perception and experience – the first-person perspective. It is the alive, thinking, feeling 'you' as a whole, from the inside out.

In today's world, somatics has become a broad umbrella term that is used to describe different modalities or practices which encompass this internal, sensing and person-centred approach.

Not surprisingly, many of these are movement or bodywork based, or therapies which focus on the embodied experience. The mind-body connection.

In somatic therapies the client is an active and engaged participant. It isn't a passive or receiving therapy like a massage. It's done with you, not done to you.

From this broad field of somatics, our focus in this book is on somatic movement education.

What is somatic movement education?

The aim by the end of this book is that you will have the experience of what somatic movement education is about – and is about for you. As it offers both a movement-based system and an educational process.

The chapters ahead will go into detail on how this works. But if you are coming across this modality for the first time then somatic movement education describes a system of sensory-motor training that is designed to create change and awareness from the inside out.

It uses gentle and specific movements to help teach the brain and body how to release habits and patterns of muscular holding.

Rather than spot fixing a problem, it aims to address the underlying presentation through the postural habits and patterns of movement that can be contributing to ongoing tightness and restriction.

Somatic movement education is an effective to way to offset tight muscles, reduce pain, improve posture and find a sense of freedom and ease of movement.

It is intelligent movement. The smart muscles, smart brain way.

The framework of somatic movement education is informed by the work of the late Thomas Hanna (founder of Hanna Somatics) along with other somatic educators before and after. You might also hear it called Clinical Somatics, Clinical Somatic Education, and even just Somatics for short.

What makes it different to many other movement modalities is the emphasis on 'education.'

You come away with practical, empowering movement tools to keep using. These are an effective and gentle reset for the brain and body. A reminder of our relaxed potential.

It also doesn't seek to replace or take away from the activities you like to do. It is about how we can keep doing the things we love to do, for as long as possible (or in some cases, to get back to them).

The somatic movement exercises can be learnt as a standalone movement practice – as we will learn the foundations of here in this book. They can also form important self-care for clients between their clinical somatic sessions. In a clinical session, a practitioner has been trained to offer hands-on techniques, along with the movements, tailored to the individual and their presenting patterns.

As with anything new and requiring internal change, it can feel a lot to remember when first learning. Having companion guide resources, like this book, offers additional support.

Small movements done consistently becomes the change.

But before we start moving, let's look at how those muscles can become tight and stay tight. And why stretching doesn't always help...

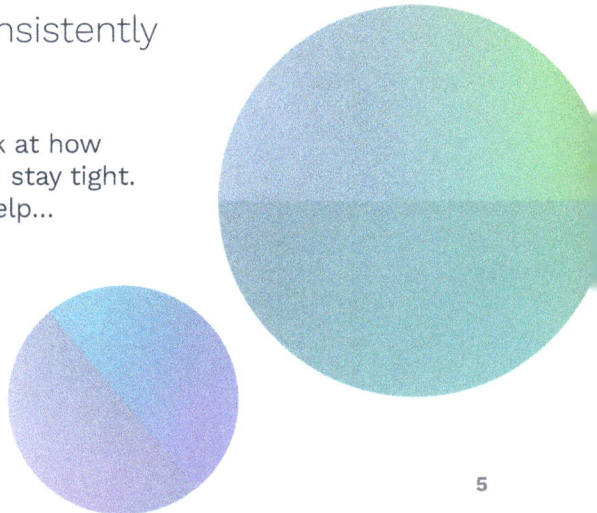

Understanding posture and patterns

How did we get here?
Why muscles become tight... and stay tight

Habits. Habits. Habits

The science and study of habits is a feature in many different areas today, from business and productivity practices to optimising performance and personal development. When it comes to our muscles and movement patterns, then the principles around habits are no different.

What fires together, wires together

Without our brain, our muscular-skeletal system wouldn't move at all. Our muscles are not inherently smart. They need the rest of us. We operate and coordinate as a system, together.

Our muscles need our brain

Once we've learnt movement patterns, and repeat them, repeatedly, then they can become automatic. It's why we can wake up each day without having to learn how to walk all over again. It just happens automatically and we don't need to think about it. We can use our energy and focus for other tasks, like what to do that day.

Habits come about through repetition

You might be someone that sits at desk for hours at a time, or hunched over a keyboard or device. You might be picking up and carrying a small child on one hip, or play a sport or musical instrument that's dominant to one side. There could have been a time or an event where you had to modify how you moved like after an accident, an injury, surgery or illness.

We all have and hold our unique life histories and experiences. Just as the saying goes that 'we are creatures of habit,' we are also **postures of habit**.

When our muscles experience a constant repetition of a pattern, or there's a state of contraction, tightness, holding on and this isn't offset, changed or reset in anyway then it can become a habit. It can become the 'new normal.' It starts running on autopilot, in the background – sometimes all the time.

Our brain doesn't distinguish if a habit is good or bad, helpful or unhelpful – it's more like, *Oh you're doing a lot of this, let me help, I'll take over, store it and run it in the background so you don't have to think about it anymore.*

It becomes unconscious and is happening out of our awareness.

We might not even know or feel our own patterns of muscular holding and contraction – well perhaps not until something like pain, discomfort or restriction starts to creep in. Then we say that 'something is getting in our way.' Without considering it could be us that has become the way. And we might not associate a new pain in the shoulder, to an old pain that was far away, like a past ankle injury. But the conditions may have begun a long time ago. It can also be confounding when the pain isn't always where the problem is.

It is repetition that becomes us. That becomes our posture. That becomes our areas of tightness and holding.

Unless we get some new information, some inputs, so that our sensory-motor system can notice and recalibrate, then we are going to keep remembering and reinforcing a pattern as normal.

It is why when someone says to 'pull your shoulders back,' you can draw them back and make that happen, but they won't naturally stay back. As soon as you stop trying or thinking them back they will return to their previous position – where the brain and body perceives is the resting 'normal.'

In Thomas Hanna's work to describe how this habituation can occur, he coined the term **Sensory Motor Amnesia** (or SMA) and emphasised that it is a process that requires education, rather than treatment. To learn or relearn what has been forgotten, the muscle memory.

When a movement pathway is running on autopilot then it needs a deliberate and conscious pattern disruptor.

Luckily there is a movement system designed to do this. Enter our somatic movements and a process called pandiculation. Let's take a look at this next, as often when people realise they have something they want to change they do the opposite, like trying to stretch those rounded shoulders back into place. But stretching isn't going to create long-term habit change. Let's see why.

Pandiculation

The smart way to create change

When we think about a tight muscle our first instinct is probably to 'give it a bit of a stretch.' Because we want to feel something different. We want to try to offset. And we may even get some temporary relief.

There's nothing wrong with stretching or with wanting to stretch. It's just that stretching doesn't always educate the brain in the way we need to create real change, to create the underlying habit change.

In passive stretching we can often engage or evoke the stretch reflex. This is an automatic and protective response that happens very fast, at the level of the spinal cord. It sends the message signals to 'act now and contract' so we don't cause injury or tearing.

You've probably experienced this before if you've taken a stretch a little too far, or maybe even felt the consequences of that the next day.

The stretch reflex is a quick and protective response. There isn't time for it to travel all the way up to the parts of the brain to process and have a discussion about what's going on.

From my own experience, I also learnt that it's pretty tricky to try to stretch (an already) tight muscle. Where is it going to go? If we can't sense and access the relaxed resting potential, then pulling against something tight can be counter-productive. It could even contract more in response.

It's a bit like the image of untangling a ball of string, if we yank on the one loose thread, then we get nowhere fast, it just becomes a harder knot to untangle, and that will take us more time.

Interestingly, tight muscles can also mean tired muscles, because it takes energy to maintain a state of contraction and holding (even if we don't consciously sense it). For some people, that might actually feel, or be perceived, like it's a weak muscle that needs strengthening, when in some cases it's a muscle that is strongly holding on. What it needs is education to release the underlying tightness and habituation.

Rather than strengthening existing patterns, if we learn to first consciously release then we have access to our full range, control and potential. This is supple strength.

How do we do this?

Well if stretching doesn't teach or create lasting change for our tight muscles and habit patterns, then we need an alternative.

This is where somatic movement education offers a different approach. It has the opposite approach to stretching.

It is about creating a connection and conversation between the brain and muscle or the group of moving muscles.

This happens through the sensory-motor system, the part of brain that coordinates sensing and moving together.

Remembering that for a habit to change, like a tight group of muscles or a movement pathway, it requires a deliberate, conscious pattern disrupter.

Somatic movement education does this by applying the principles of pandiculation to movement patterns.

Pandiculation might sound like a big word, but you've likely seen this in action before, especially if you have a cat or a dog.

The pandicular response is easily observed in animals – and we do it too, it's that yawn-like movement that occurs on waking, or after being still or stationary for a long time.

It is getting the nervous system and all of us online, ready to move. A reset of where the brain and muscles are at.

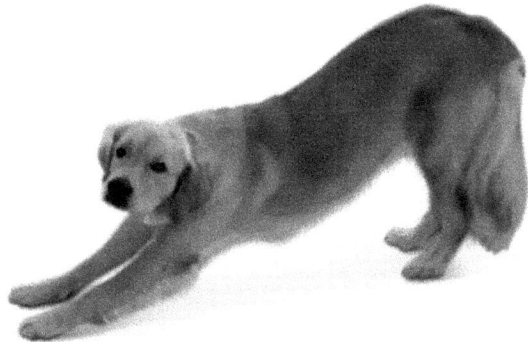

Animals do it a lot. And babies too. But us adults, well we could use some more of it. The good news is that this is what our somatic movements are helping us to do.

This means that after sitting for hours at a desk we don't have to take those hunched, tight, rounded shoulders – the habituation – into the rest of the day or night. Instead, we can pandiculate using specific somatic movements so that the brain and body have the opportunity to remember and return to neutral, a place of non-effort. To offset and reset.

To do this, a somatic movement will often comprise three parts, or phases within it. Just like a story book, our movements have a beginning, a middle and an end phase:

1] Move into pattern

First, we're going to move into the pattern. We're going to **do more of what the brain already wants to do,** like rounding the shoulders inwards. Instead of stretching and forcing the shoulders back we are consciously creating the pattern and contracting inwards. Now the brain can sense and feel what 'tight' is really like. We've turned the volume up so to speak.

2] Slow release out

Next we have our slow, controlled release out. This is about mindful movement. It is **where the learning and reset can happen.** The brain is sensing and coordinating the motor movement which allows us to discover the full range and control of our muscles and movement pathways. We're slowly dialling the volume back, listening to every part (or noticing the places that skip). We are learning where our relaxed baseline can actually be. Those shoulders may now find that they can rest further back and the chest naturally opens.

3] Integrating pause

Then a relaxed integrating pause. A moment of rest and stillness for the **learning to absorb,** for the brain and body and our nervous system to notice, sense and feel into any changes we've made. The macro and the micro, because we are an interconnected whole. As those shoulders sit back with new found ease we may be able to breathe more fully, or the neck feels relaxed. Take time to notice what you notice.

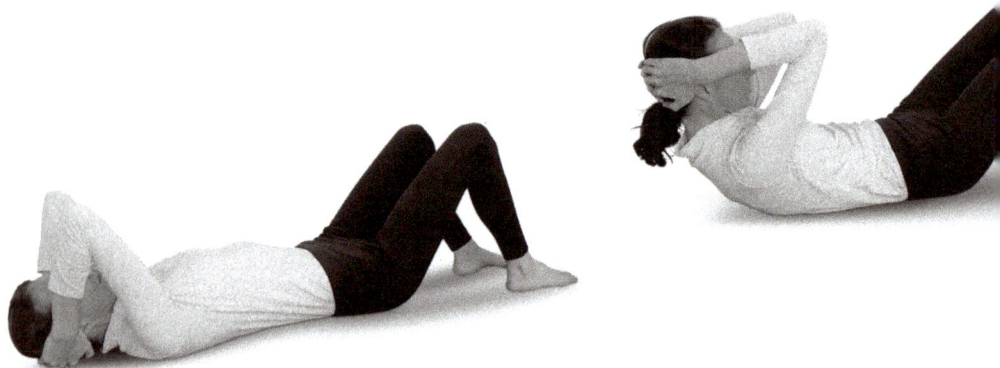

What somatic movement education is aiming to do is apply the principles of pandiculation to voluntary movement. This engages the sensory-motor part of the brain, our nervous system and the kinetic chains that move our muscular-skeletal system.

Here is our 'education.'

Rather than stretching against a tight muscle, we are consciously learning (or unlearning) what contraction or tight really is. And then coordinating a slow mindful release to be able to sense and feel the full range, control and potential of those once tight muscles.

Remembering that when a movement pathway has been running on autopilot then it needs a deliberate and conscious pattern disruptor. Which is what pandiculation and somatic movements can do.

It's mindful, intelligent movement.

It's the smart muscles, smart brain way.

And because it's about recognising that we are a whole, interconnected, coordinating, moving system then we will rarely focus on one muscle in isolation.

Instead we look at our patterns of movement, our posture and the adaptations to stress and where habituation can commonly occur. Because as humans we share some predictable patterns.

Let's take a look at these somatic patterns next, as it's going to help inform our movement practice ahead.

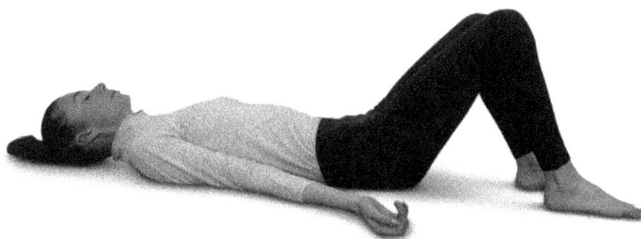

Somatic posture patterns

The patterns of being human

The somatic postural patterns and adaptations of being human.

We've learnt how those tight muscles can come about and stay about (habits and repetition) and what needs to start to happen to create some real change (education, such as pandiculation instead of stretching).

But how do we know what movements to do, when and why? How do we apply this to ourselves?

The power and benefit within somatic movements is in how they correspond to postural and movement patterns. You could call these somatic patterns, or just the result of being human.

These are universal, reflex-like responses or predictable patterns that we can see present through the front, back and sides of the body. It is about how we might adapt to stress and the activities of life, and where we then hold that habituation.

As we've learned, it is not so much whether a stress is good or bad, an event negative or positive, it is simply about the repetition that becomes us. We need to be able to move into patterns and to respond to life, but we also need to be able to move out of them, fully.

Let's take an overview of the somatic responses and postural presentations for the front, back and sides of the body. The corresponding movement sections ahead will then go into further detail as we apply theory to movement.

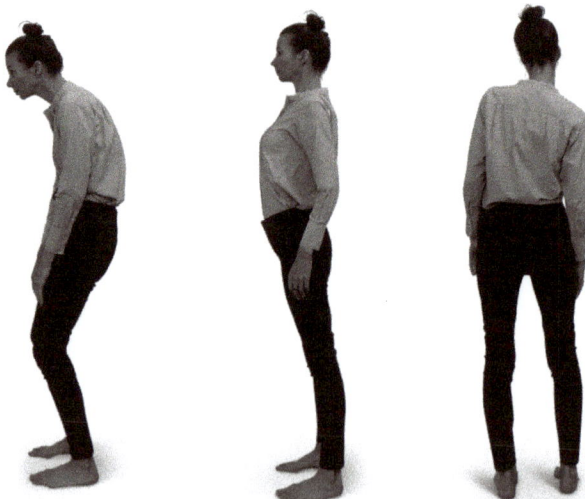

Exercise: Take photos

Know Thyself

Before we start to look at how these somatic responses and muscle imbalances can appear, a useful exercise is to first take some full-length photos of yourself in standing, from the front, back and both sides of the body.

Allow yourself to stand naturally, without holding, forcing or trying to create a posture. The aim is just to see how your brain and body is organising itself right now.

If no one is nearby to help take the photos then you can prop a phone/camera up and record yourself turning and pausing at each of the four areas: front on, back of the body and both sides.

This is just for you to see and have as a baseline – a before picture. This can be helpful to have as you move through the book and continue your somatic movement practice.

You may also like to make a note of the date you took this and reflect on any goals you have.

- Perhaps there's an activity you'd like to get back to...
- Or to wake up with (or get through the day) with less tension, less pain.
- It might be about ageing well and moving through life well.
- It could be about finding tools to help manage a condition.
- Or a curiosity about a different way of moving, an embodied practice, to level-up and optimise (smart body and brain).

You might also jot down any past events, like an accident, a broken bone or sprain, an injury, surgery or illness, along with the approximate year.

Having a baseline, a before picture and reflection can give some interesting insight into our unique patterns and habits.

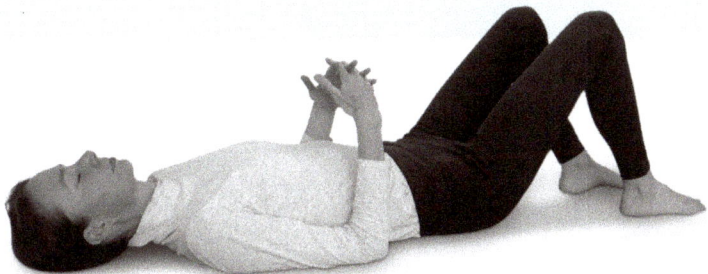

Front of the body

Rounded shoulders, forward head, tech neck

For the front of the body, the somatic posture patterns relate to muscles and movement that brings us into forward flexion, a curling or rounding inwards.

This can feel like a familiar movement or comforting position, as it is one we've known since being in the womb.

It also links with the early startle response seen in newborns. As adults, we retain aspects of this reflex-like protective impulse.

If you think about being startled or when you've had a fright then this contraction happens automatically, reflexively, to round and protect us and the many important organs vulnerable to exposure.

The muscles through the front of the torso and pelvis contract to pull us into a flexed, curved position.

The energy is stop, withdraw, protect and become small.

It is an important evolutionary response. But once the perceived danger, or the trigger has passed, we also need to be able to come out of this contraction. To offset and reset.

For the front of the body, the somatic holding patterns and posture picture will often mirror the same rounding into flexion of this familiar, full-body movement.

It was once a visual associated more with older age, the hunched, stooped posture.

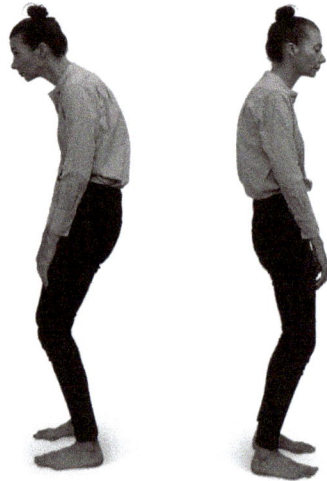

Yet with our modern technology we are now actively adopting this posture at any age as we spend hours sitting and curling over devices, desks, keyboards, and steering wheels.

It has become the rounded shoulders, forward head or 'tech neck' posture.

As it is our habits – the repetition over time – that become us.

It is a postural picture where you might hear (or be told) 'just stand up straight and pull your shoulders back.' Which is what you then try to do, to pull the shoulders back, or even lean back. But without effort, those shoulders are not going to stay back. As soon as we stop trying, or thinking about it, the old patterns will return. The brain and body has a different program, or baseline understanding, that it is operating from. What those shoulders really need is some gentle education. A reminder of their resting relaxed potential rather than a state of constant contraction – especially if we work in this position for hours and days at a time.

Our habits don't discriminate with age.

Posture problems are not just for 'when we get old,' nor do they need to be an inevitable sign of ageing.

But we do need the movement tools to help us manage life.

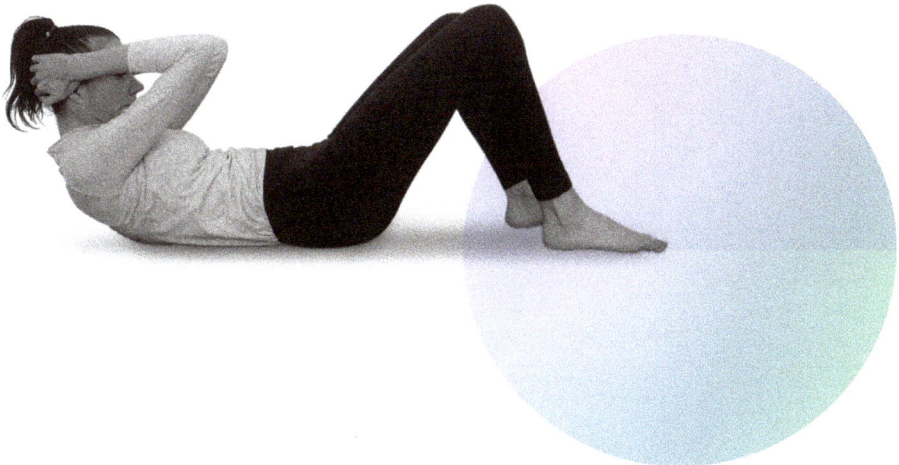

Back of the body

Upright, ready, on, go go go...

The opposite of flexion and withdrawal through the front is the action and extension we can see (and often feel) through the back of the body. That which keeps us upright, standing to attention and readies us for forward motion.

If the front was stop, then the back is go. Red light, green light.

However if these back extensor muscles are constantly being held in a state of contraction, like we are always on and ready (just in case) then it wouldn't be surprising to start to hear complaints of a tight or sore or tired back.

It is a somatic posture picture of standing ready to attention, ready to spring into action.

We might also see what people call a 'sway back.' This is the forward tilt that occurs as the muscles of the lower back contract and shorten. This lordotic curve sends the abdomen forwards in front. The problem becomes when these back muscles are always on, even when they don't need to be, like when we're lying down at rest.

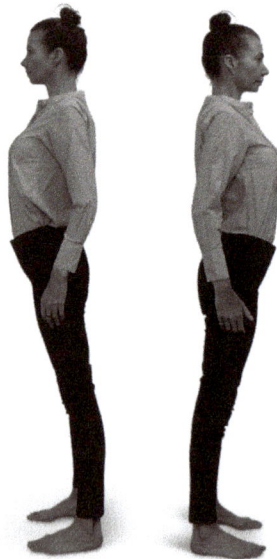

The yoga class from hell

I will never forget being in a yoga teacher training class that was focusing on strengthening and core work. I was really struggling. I couldn't seem to coordinate the movement or when I did, I couldn't hold it. After more than a year of this training was my core really that weak?

I looked around at my fellow students that were effortlessly moving and felt the rising panic that I couldn't do this and I didn't know why.

The instructor came past me and tapped the space on the floor under my lower back to indicate this was the problem. Lying down my lower back didn't rest on the floor. It wasn't even near the floor. It arched up like a small tunnel you could drive a truck through.

But I couldn't change this. Not back then. To get my lower back down I would need to recruit and use a variety of other unhelpful and uncomfortable strategies. I left that class feeling like a failure.

Why was this not getting easier? Why did it hurt so much? Why didn't massage or physical therapies help? What was I doing wrong? Maybe I shouldn't be a yoga teacher...

Now, what I would tell myself is that it's pretty hard to engage the core – the front of the body – when the back is already on and working. It's like having your foot on the brake and accelerator at the same time. What I needed was to go back a step. To ground zero and to reset the canvas. I needed to be able to coordinate the front and back working together. To teach my body and brain what is relaxed and what is contracted. To find and feel neutral and from there be able to move and actually strengthen.

If I was in that class today, with what I know now, those movements would pose no issue.

Sometimes the problem isn't always where or what we think it is. It's knowing the smart muscles, smart brain way.

We need all of us

It is important to remember that as part of being human, we need all of these responses – front and back, to stop and go. One pattern or posture picture isn't better or more desirable than the other. We need the ability to access and move into them when life requires us to. But equally we need to be able come out of them, so it doesn't become an unconscious holding habit. We can see this too with the sides of the body.

Sides of the body

Uneven posture, alignment issues, accidents and injuries

The sides of the body and particularly the muscles of the waist influence our postural symmetry and how we counter-balance.

Just as we've looked at the front-back dynamic, we also have a side-to-side relationship.

'Wow, I have one arm longer than the other,' said the client, an artist, as he looked from the mirror to me, back to the mirror and me again.

'Yes,' I said. 'It appears that way, but let's look at the waist.'

Visible through the same side waist was a curve, a contraction of the muscles to this side. The arm appeared longer in response to this shortening and sideways cringe.

The client had mentioned a leg injury that happened a long time ago, but that wasn't the problem now, the pain was in the arm and shoulder...

When we experience a one-sided event like an accident or an injury then there's a postural change that happens – usually a cringe or curve to one side as we protect, guard and try to move away from pain or further injury.

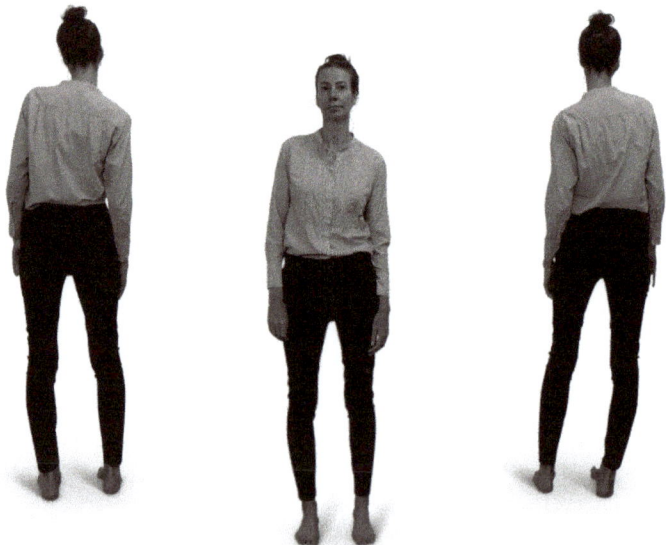

If you've ever sprained an ankle then you'll remember how you had to shift your weight off that leg and modify how you moved for a while. It is a necessary accommodation to avoid pain and further damage. In order to make this adjustment happen, the muscles of the waist have to respond. And so that we then stay as upright as possible (and not just topple over to one side) other compensatory patterns occur to counterbalance us. A righting response, like a zig-zag through our posture.

At the time we need this. But as we know can happen with repetition, the patterns of muscular contraction could still be holding in the centre of the body, long after the ankle has healed.

Years later we might not associate any new pains, or problems with that old injury, particularly if they arise elsewhere, like the shoulder and arm. However, the conditions, the holding and habits may have been set in motion a long time ago.

It doesn't always have to begin with a sudden, major event or accident. In its subtle form the repetition of everyday activities we do to one side can also contribute to patterns of muscular imbalance. We might be picking up and carrying a small child on one hip, or carrying a heavy bag over one shoulder, or playing a sport or musical instrument that favours one side.

It is the habit, the repetition, that can become us if we don't have the tools to offset and reset.

In our posture this may show up as shoulders or hips that appear uneven, visually different arm or leg lengths, the head and neck tilting to one side. We may start trying to address all these individual differences separately, to spot fix them, without ever addressing or considering the muscles of the side waist.

It is also a concept that is useful to keep in mind when considering pain – as in some cases the pain isn't always where the problem originates from.

We need to take in the whole context, the whole of you.

Remembering in somatic movement education, it is not about targeting one muscle in isolation, but how we organise ourselves as a system. It is like conducting the orchestra within and of your body. It's just that sometimes we may not all be playing together, or in tune.

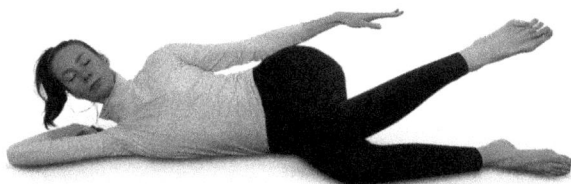

Our function affects our structure

When there is a sustained muscular contraction and patterns of imbalance occurring through the torso, it can start to impact important structures, like our spine. People might even be told they have a functional scoliosis or non-structural scoliosis. This is where there is a side-to-side curve or pull through the spine but the origins are coming from something like muscular imbalances.

The good news is we have a system of sensory-motor education to help repattern and support our overall function. We can apply specific movements to patterns, moving into and out of them, somatically.

Competing patterns, mixed patterns, our unique patterns

It is unlikely that we are ever 'just one' pattern.

If only it was that simple! But in reality we are all the patterns. As such, we might have combinations of them or different areas of tightness and holding occurring at the same time.

For example, a forward head and neck position and a sway back. The shoulders and upper chest might be contracting and rounding us inwards while at the same time the lower back is contracting and arching to send us forwards. Front and Back, Stop and Go. Like an accelerator and brake trying to work at the same time.

We could also be rounding inwards with a side twist, or arching back with it. We might go from being 'on' all day through the back to sinking and collapsing through front to switch off when we finally get to stop. Only to repeat it the next day when the alarm clock or coffee kicks us into gear.

There is also the energetics of how we feel on the inside versus how we move and present to the world.

While the somatic patterns, the full body responses of the front, back and sides go with being human, how we as the human develop and habituate into them is going to be unique to us.

We will all have our individual tendencies that reflect our habits, patterns, stressors, experiences and adaptations. Our life.

Identifying patterns within ourselves doesn't need to be another thing we have to feel bad about or instantly fix. It is just information and we can use it to help guide our movement practice ahead and to tailor it to what presents for us.

This is somatic wisdom – what it is to really know ourselves, from the inside out and to support this 'home' of ours that has carried us thus far.

Exercise: Revisit photos

If you did the exercise and took pictures of yourself in standing, and reflected on any past injuries or events, then this is a good time to review.

- Can you visually see any patterns through the front, the back and the sides of your body?
- Do you notice any areas of imbalance, like arm length difference, shoulders that appear uneven, or a tilt of the head and neck? We might see clothing bunch and gather differently, like around the waist. Side-on we might notice the head jutting forward and the shoulders rounding, or that the shoulders are pulled back to attention.
- Sometimes it is not so much what we see visually but our feeling sense from within, or what is occurring in life right now. We might know that we have a deadline and have to be on, or that we've felt more withdrawn lately.

Remember it is both the sensory and the motor, what we sense and how we feel is equally important to consider along with how we physically move, hold and organise ourselves.

Importantly, there's no judgement that goes with this. It is just information.

There can be many reasons as to why and how our posture has come about. We want to approach all our somatic movement work with a playful, gentle, kind curiosity. This is also the optimal state for learning and to create change.

It can be a useful exercise to revisit pictures and movement goals over time. What does our posture look like before a practice and after? What is it like after a month, or three months, or a year from now? And how do we actually feel in ourselves. Was there an activity that we were able to get back to?

Developmental perspective

Linking our early sensory-motor development

It can be easy to forget that we didn't just arrive into these fully grown adult bodies. We had to develop into them.

We had to learn how to move, for our muscles to form, and our motor patterns to connect. Then to repeat them, over and over again.

You could say our habits began a long time ago!

When we arrive in the world as a newborn, we start out as a helpless bundle of reflexes. During the first year to 18 months, as we develop to become a two-legged explorer, the building blocks of our sensory-motor system are forming. A sort of blueprint of our development ahead. Each stage is laying the foundations and milestones for the next phase to come.

The way I approach and teach somatic movement is to interweave a developmental perspective.

This came about as I became curious based on my work with babies and children and then separately, what I was seeing in some adult clients learning somatic movement for the first time. I had questions.

What if it's not always sensory-motor amnesia and a habit dysfunction that's occurred as adults ... what if for some people the patterns started from our early months or years of development?

As when we're an infant, our motor development is occurring like step-by-step building blocks. A layering of phases for what is to come.

What if it's not always that a sensory-motor pathway or movement pattern was forgotten, but that it was not learnt or clearly defined early on?

Of course, by the time we're in adult bodies asking this, it can be hard to know. Which is why keeping a developmental perspective alongside can be both helpful and, in some cases, necessary.

Even if we can't go back in time, we can still connect the phases of early sensory-motor development with our somatic movement education practice. This is why it is part of the smart muscles, smart brain way.

There may be some that argue that it doesn't matter how we got to here as long as we got here. Humans are creative, adaptable creatures, and children especially so. They will find a way. But it may not always be the most efficient or optimal movement way, and requires energy to maintain.

Just because something doesn't present as an issue at the time, doesn't mean it won't have flow on affects for future development, or into our adult years.

Using and overlaying a developmental approach will help to guide the structure of our learning here. We can explore and build our somatic movement foundations through the phases of development. Thereby linking somatic movements with early sensory-motor development and the unfolding themes that are occurring for the front, back and sides of the body. It is part of the smart muscles, smart brain way.

The bendy baby

When muscle disparity begins young.

From my work with clients, from babies through to older adults, what I've observed are patterns and adaptations that can begin very early on.

One of the most striking is that of the so-called 'bendy baby.' This is the infant where we can see a postural asymmetry or imbalances appearing left and right. Characteristic is a tilt of the head and neck, with marked restriction in being able to turn the head freely, equally, to both sides. The soft plates of the head may appear misshapen or flatter on one side and in response the level of the eyeline and forehead may seem uneven. The flow on for the rest of the body is that it can appear 'bendy', rather than straight or symmetrical. In my training this was called KISS (a Kinematic Imbalance due to Suboccipital Strain).

A restriction in the upper cervical spine (the neck area) is not uncommon in newborns, particularly as the journey to be born places a lot of pressure on this area. This restriction will often resolve early on and through activities like tummy-time which encourages the neck to mobilise.

But if this does not resolve in the early months, if the restriction remains and becomes fixed, then these conditions can contribute to a postural asymmetry, an imbalance that all the sensory-motor building blocks and milestones to come are then working from. As the centre, the midline axis (head, neck, body), is not straight or symmetrical to begin with. It isn't a true sense of centre. It is developing from disparity and the muscles and posture will reflect this.

The bendy baby may become the child or adult with scoliosis or other postural issues arising from this early imbalance.

Creating your movement practice

Setting up a mindful, sustainable movement practice

Things to keep in mind before and during a movement practice:

- **Move gently, slowly, using mindful awareness**
  It is about quality over quantity

- **Never force a movement or move into pain**
  Avoid going into stretch sensations (ease back a bit)

- **Movements can be small, incremental**
  They can even be visualised

- **Rest and relax after completing a movement and in-between repetitions**
  Allow the brain and body time to integrate
  Take this time to notice and sense

- **Patience and positivity**
  It can take time to change long-held patterns

- **To approach with a playful, gentle curiosity and non-judgemental awareness**
  We learn best when we're not stressed

- **Consistency of practice**
  For as long as we have a body then these movements can apply.

Do I need special equipment?

No, just yourself. You are the special equipment.

Wear comfortable clothing you can move in (remove belts and avoid tight jeans or clothing that restricts movement).

When to practise?

The best time to practise is when you have, or can make the time. For some people it will be the morning, for others the evening, or it may be the middle of the day when the kids are at school. Find a rhythm that works for you.

The morning can help set us up for the day and offset any pretzel-like sleeping habits. The evening can help unwind the accumulated tension of the day and take a relaxed body to bed, meaning we don't have to take those rounded shoulders or tight back into the night.

Where to practise?

The floor is your friend. In this book our focus is on movements that are floor-based or that you can do on a firm surface, like an exercise table. The firm surface provides neuro-feedback, or clear information to the brain as it senses and feels where the body is. If we use a soft squishy surface like a mattress, we can sink into it, and we might be sinking into imbalanced patterns as there isn't a clear level stop.

In this sense, the floor is optimal (and generally available) and you can make it comfortable with exercise mats or a blanket beneath.

A distraction free space (as much as possible).

Somatic movement is mindful movement. To focus the part of the brain where we need to create muscle and movement change (the sensory-motor cortex) then we don't want to be multi-tasking and engaging other areas of our brain, like listening to music, a podcast, having the tv on, the 'help' of a pet, or thinking about what to have for lunch or our to-do list.

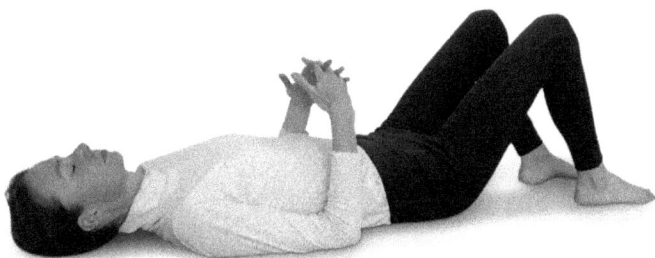

The power of visualisation

Science has studied and demonstrated the power of visualisation and the impact on motor pathways. The act of visualising a movement, imagining it, practising it and seeing it in your mind, helps to forge the motor pathways and connections as if you were actually moving. It is a performance technique used in sport, in music, in injury recovery.

Where your focus goes, your attention and pathways grow. What fires together, wires together.

In somatic movement, this makes motor planning – the act of visualising yourself coordinating and completing a movement – a powerful tool to use. It is also makes these movements accessible. This is something that you can do in bed!

Visualising movements can be very useful when first learning. You might read or listen to the instructions first and then put it into motion in your mind.

A helpful way to incorporate visualisation in your practice is to use motor planning as the first step. Before you even start moving, start by planning it in your mind. Go through the entire movement, seeing it in your mind. Then the next time start to initiate the movement and grow incrementally.

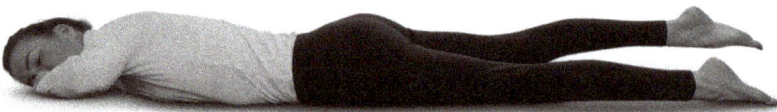

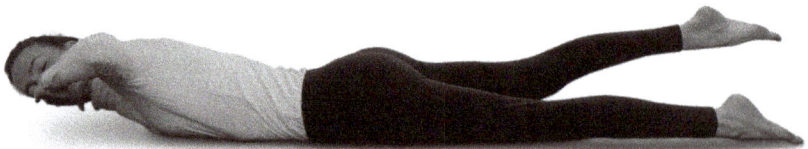

Growing a movement

It can be tempting to see how far we can go in a movement, to see how big we can make it. We might really want to *feel* some sort of sensation. But if we go from 0 to 100 we can often miss the middle, and we might also be moving really fast to get there.

Slowing down and breaking down a movement incrementally can help us notice more. To sense and feel more. To ultimately change more. And to move safely.

Growing a movement incrementally benefits the body and the brain. It is also a safe way to move. It lets us feel our capacity and range on any given day.

Having visualised a movement first you might then begin to initiate the movement.

• Start by letting the connections begin to engage and then change your mind and ease back.
• The next time you might explore moving into the movement 10%, notice, then release out.
• Then the next time 30%, 50% and so on.

In somatic movement there isn't an end goal, a final posture or shape that you must accomplish.

There is just what is there for you, and that may change day-to-day.

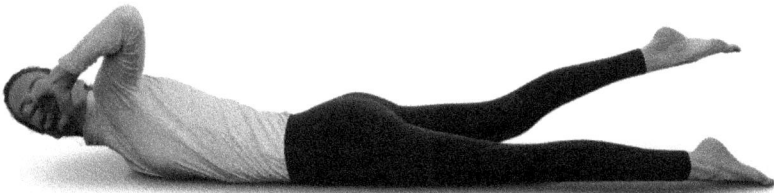

How many repetitions?

The idea of 'repetitions' is a concept that sits in the exercise and fitness world.

While these movements often get called 'exercises' they are really 'explorations.'

You are exploring a movement.

Explorations invite curiosity. Perhaps we start small, just beginning a movement, then the next time we move a little further.

As I say to my clients, I would much rather they do three slow conscious explorations than a set number just to go through the motions.

While you will find repetition suggestions along with each movement it is important to remember that this is not a mechanical, isolated, exercise. It is all of you coordinating this movement, from the inside out.

Pushing our nervous system to learn or change all at once is also counterproductive.

On some days we will have more or less capacity.

Part of developing our somatic wisdom is to know what we need and when, and to listen to the body.

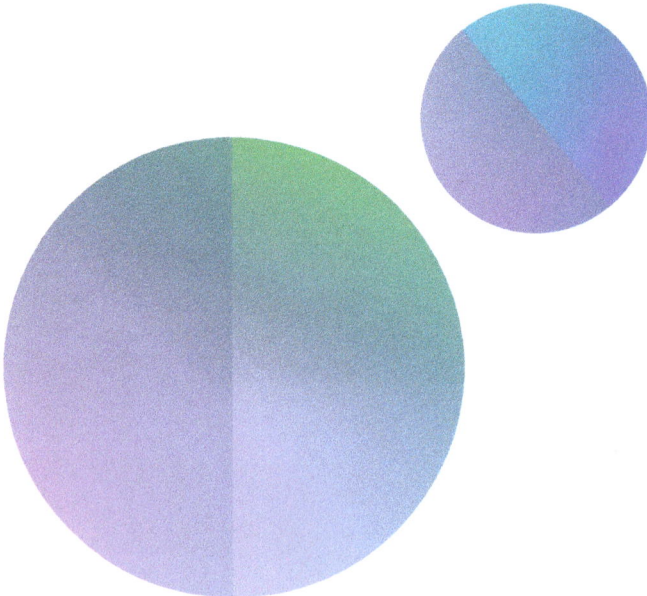

Pacing and Progression: starting where you are at

The movements in this book are set out in a progressive way, layering the unfolding phases of early movement development, so that you can build solid foundations for your somatic movement practice.

While the learning structure is offered in this way, the pace of learning is up to you.

The pace is guided by you – as we all start where we are at and in the body we are in.

Our physical home is the sum of all our life experiences and journeys. If we've had accidents, injuries, illness or events along the way, we may be going at a different pace.

There will be some people that can explore all the movements in this book in one session and others that may take a section, or even one movement, week by week. It may also form a reference guide, to check back in as clients do alongside their clinical sessions.

At the end of the book you will find sequence suggestions for putting these movements together for different focus areas, as well as shorter or longer practice options.

It can also be helpful to remember that because we are consciously sensing and coordinating movement (brain-based movement) we can feel quite mentally tired from these exercises – we can feel 'brain tired' even though our focus was on moving the body.

Just as the body holds our unique life experiences, the issues and (muscle) tissues can often weave together. If any movement practice brings strong sensations to the surface, then it is a good idea to be working alongside appropriate therapists. To have your support team. Somatic movements can be a helpful integration tool alongside other talk-based therapies.

But there is no one right pace for learning and pushing through doesn't create change faster.

Our desire or will for change must match the pace with which we can integrate as a whole.

Small inputs (movements) done consistently create the underlying habit change.

Do I have to keep practising?

Practice as a choice, not a chore.

One of the reasons I share this work is that I believe somatic movements help to bring joy back into movement (and life!) – the sense of play and wonder that pain can constrict out of us.

These are movements that you get to do, not have to do. But they are also never one and done. Just as you ate a meal yesterday, it doesn't mean you won't eat again today or tomorrow.

It's like brushing teeth, but for movement maintenance. For body and mind.

For as long as we have a body and are in relation with life then we will be interacting with the somatic responses (the patterns of the front, back and sides of the body). We will be accumulating stress and tension, and cementing habits and patterns.

Our habits and grooves can run deep. I know if I don't do my somatic movement practice regularly then old patterns that twist and pull will start to creep in. What is familiar is comfortable, even if it creates a physical discomfort.

Somatic movements offer a gentle reminder of a different possibility.

It is a reminder that only works if we use it.

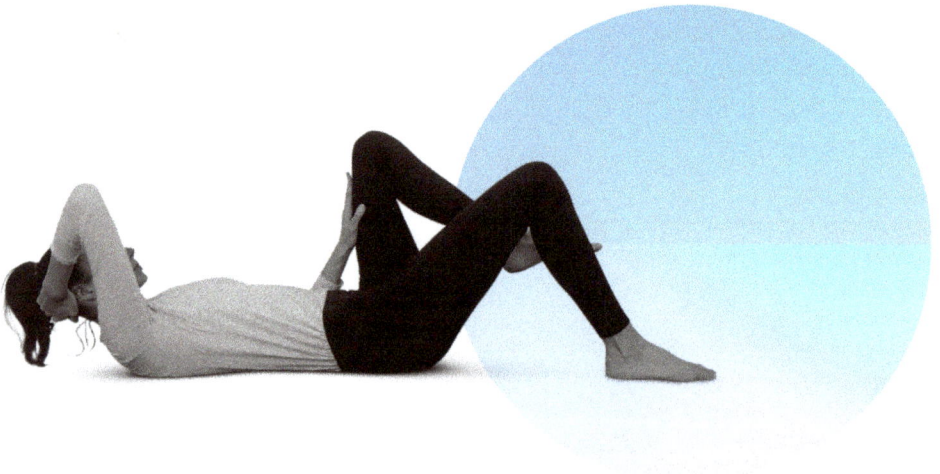

When will I notice change?

To create change fast, we first have to slow down.

Slowing down to speed up.

I know from my own experience that pain is an incredible motivator. You just want it gone. For some people this will take them on a path of exploration, while others might be looking for a quick fix.

I see this spectrum often in clinic. It is not uncommon for people to find or try somatics as a last resort. Usually because they've tried everything else and there's nothing to lose. Sometimes these clients are highly motivated to practise movements between sessions, other times not. Sometimes people will come once just to check it out or because they want a quick and easy fix, or they want the practitioner to do the work for them.

The irony with somatic movements is that, in time, they do offer a quick fix. But to get there fast, we first have to slow down.

As you'll see by the end of this book, you'll have movement tools to offset activities like sitting at a desk all day, or to wind down the back tension from a deadline you've been working on.

In the beginning it takes time to learn, or unlearn, or relearn movement patterns and pathways.

We may have developed a pain or problem over decades and now we are rewiring or laying new tracks that are unfamiliar. There could be known structural issues that we can't change but we can work to support our overall function ahead.

There are so many variables in how we use our body, what activities we do, and our experiences in life.

If every day we take a forest walk using the same path underfoot then it becomes clear and defined. We don't even need to think about it. But if we have to find a new route to walk then in the beginning it may not be so familiar and clear. It will take time and repetition until it becomes the new path way.

What I as the practitioner can do, is offer the information – the smart muscles, smart brain way. The movement tools and framework. The education. What I can't do is the actual movements for you.

So let's start moving!

PART ONE

Where to begin: Finding centre

centre

Starting in the centre

This first section sets up the foundations for much of the future movements to come. It is like establishing the canvas to begin exploring and moving from.

We start in the centre of the body, with our front-back relationship and our midline. Finding our centre.

Our centre is the place we move from and come back to. Often when there's a pain or problem in the extremities, like the arm, knee or foot, we look to spot fix this area. This approach might offer some relief but if we cannot connect and integrate it back to our centre, back to the rest of us, then it can be hard to hold or sustain the gains.

In somatic movement education we work from the centre out.

The first movement focuses on coordinating the front and back of the body – through the torso and the head to tail connection – moving between flexion and extension, contraction and softening.

The second movement is about rebalancing or recalibrating the first if we find we might need to. This helps to balance symmetry through the torso and our sense of a midline, our centre-line. So when we do explore other movements, or work towards the periphery, we are less likely to take pre-existing patterns of muscular holding or imbalance.

Let's start rolling.

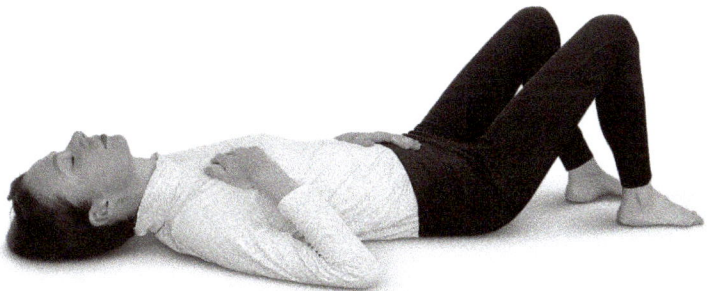

Developmental perspective

Finding our centre

When we arrive in the world as a newborn, for the first few months, we are learning what it is to have a body.

We are learning that this body has borders and boundaries to it. *Where do I begin and end, and where do you and the world around me start,* as well as being in relation to this.

Our new environment is a really different place to be after the snugness, sameness and security of the womb! It is why touch, our tactile sense, becomes so important early on and for our sensory-motor development ahead. Touch will help us to sense and feel who and where we are.

In these early months of life as we're learning we have this body, an important achievement is being able to 'find our centre' or the midline, the axis of the body.

Visually, what this looks like for an infant when lying on the back (in supine position) is the baby's head and body are aligned in the centre midline, with the hands coming together above the body at the midline and the inside of the feet also touching above. Here we have found our centre-line. Head, body, hands, feet. We have an axis!

At around three months of age an infant discovers their centre - the midline of the body - and their future axis to move from and come back to

A baby won't necessarily hold this position of 'centre' for long periods of time as they play but it is something positive to observe coming together and connecting at around three months of age.

It is this midline and symmetry that will become an important foundation for future sensory-motor development to build on (like rotation and turning). It creates an axis to move around and come back to. To be able to return to our centre when we need.

Without this idea of 'centre' we can see how the very early conditions of muscular imbalance could appear. When a postural asymmetry is present, our sense of centre is not a 'true centre.' Yet if it is all we know and can sense and feel, then it forms the baseline that our future sensory-motor building blocks begin from. Remember the bendy baby...

Our habits and patterns can start young (or be as old as we are).

I look at these beginning somatic movements as the adult equivalent of finding our centre, of recalibrating and rebalancing.

This helps to establish our foundations, the scaffolding for other movements to come. In this way, we are more likely to gain the benefits of future movements, rather than take pre-existing imbalances into them (or potentially strengthening them!)

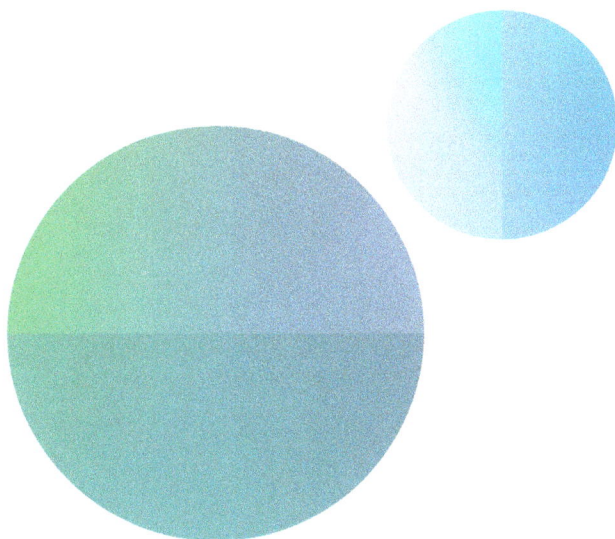

Can I do these movements in bed?

A question that often comes up is, 'can I do these movements in bed?'

For some people and situations that may be the only option, or when working just with visualisations. But ideally, we want to have a firm surface to practise on (the floor, the carpet, an exercise mat or table).

A firm surface provides neurofeedback – a clear sense to the brain of where your body is, and in relation and response to movement.

A bed is (usually) soft. So instead of a clear stop or end point in a movement, we just keep sinking.

This is the same for babies and early development. It is pretty tricky to find your centre if the surface beneath is squishy and yielding in places, compared to consistent and level.

We want to be comfortable but a firm surface is what gives feedback to the brain and body about what is moving and where.

If we want the best shot at habit change, to rewire, then a firm surface is your companion to somatic movements. The floor is your friend.

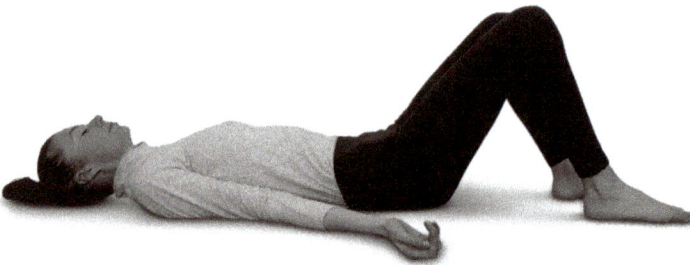

A firm surface is what gives feedback to the brain and body about what is moving and where

When to breathe?

Throughout the movement instructions you'll find guidance or movement cueing with the breath. These are just suggestions. They are suggestions on using the breath to maximise the movement pattern (eg. inhaling as you expand, exhaling as you contract). Clients often find this helpful, but the breath is unique to us.

If you need to take more breath cycles while moving then please do.

We don't want to create unnecessary tension by holding the breath, or feel like we have to speed up a movement just so we can breathe!

When you see an inhale or exhale suggested it is there as a prompt and may help moving within a pattern – but please, breathe as you need.

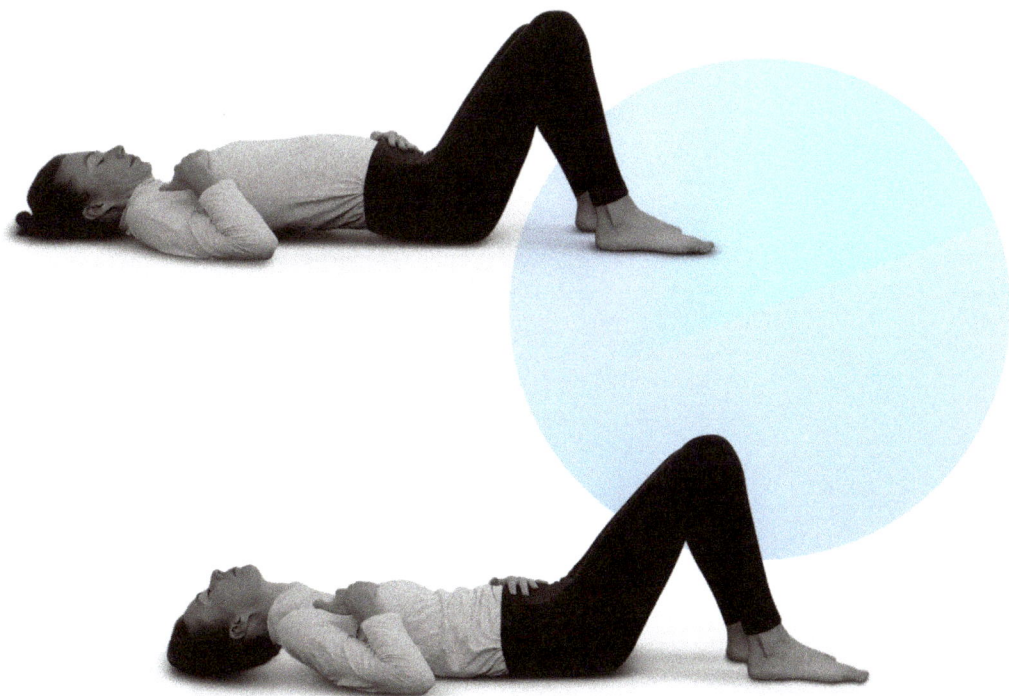

Sensing

Body Scan (to start)

Begin and end your practice with a sensing body scan.

Allow yourself to notice what is there before and what may have changed (or how it has changed) at the end.

It is like taking an inside-out snapshot.

1] Lie on your back with the arms and legs comfortably extended.

Begin by **becoming present** to your **body and breath**.

Allow your attention and awareness to turn inwards.

Notice the **points of contact** with the floor or surface beneath you.

Sense where there are gaps and arches. Is there differences or symmetry left and right?

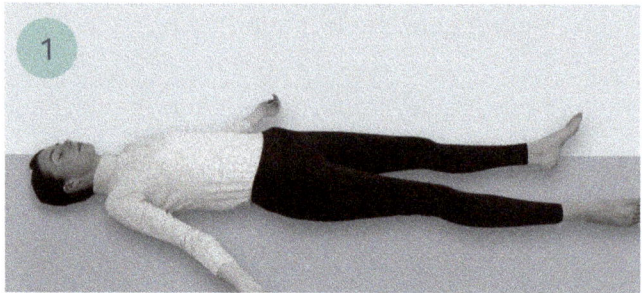

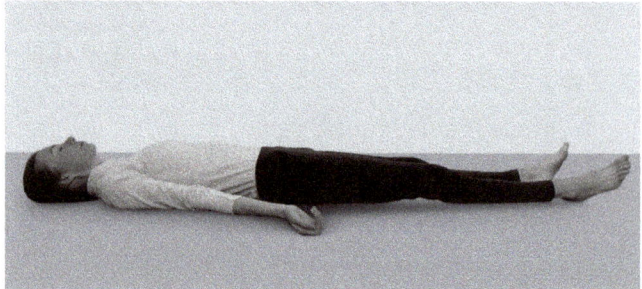

As you scan into the body you may notice

- Areas of tightness, lightness, heaviness or holding.
- Places that are easy or difficult to sense and feel.
- The symmetry or differences between left and right, any tilts or pulls to one side? Does the weight feel even through both legs? How do the feet fall?
- If there's an arch in the lower back (does one side feel higher than the other?)
- The gaps and arches that might be present around the ankles, backs of the knees, lower back, elbows, wrists, back of the neck.
- How the shoulders feel – is one side more lifted or raised, or is one more in contact with the floor?
- How the arms are arranged – do the palms rest palm up, palm down or curled around?
- The weight and place of the back of the head. You might even open the eyes and note where your gaze currently is.
- If you gently and slowly roll the head left and right, where are the natural stop points? (rather than forcing to turn)
- Where the breath flows, is it high in the chest or low in the belly? Is it shallow or deep – is there space for the breath to flow?
- If you were lying in sand what would this imprint of you look like? Capture this soft sensing internal picture. You can revisit this at the end or between movements.

Revisiting this body scan during your practice can be helpful integration time for brain and body. To sense and feel, to notice both the macro and the micro changes. What has changed and how does the whole, the whole of you, feel?

Movement 1
Finding Centre

Bringing awareness and coordination between the muscles of the front and back of the torso, as well as the head to tail connection, our midline.

This movement is traditionally known as Arch and Flatten. It is like two sides of the same coin moving together – expanding and contracting, lengthening and shortening.

Here we will explore the movement in two parts and then put it together as one wave-like movement.

Part 1 (Arch) Opening the front, contracting the back

1] Lie on your back with the **knees bent**, feet flat on the floor hip width apart, arms rest alongside the body.

Bring awareness to the breath. See if the upper chest can be quiet as you send the breath deep into the belly.

[Optional] You may like to place one **hand on the lower** belly and one on the **upper chest** for feedback as you move.

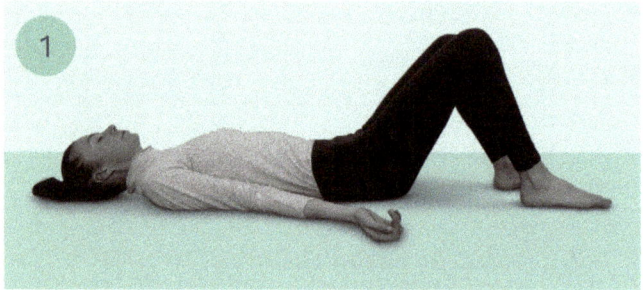

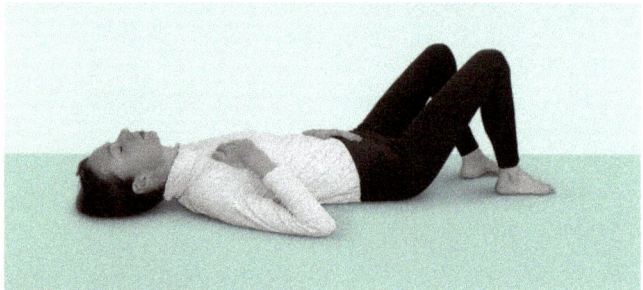

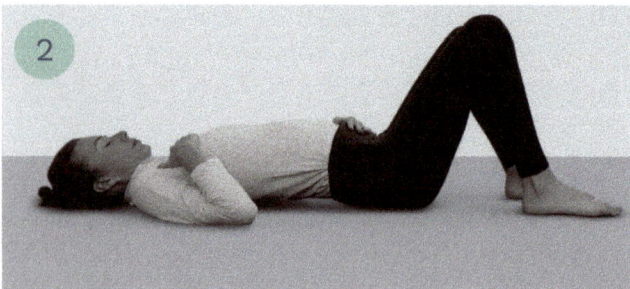

2] As you **inhale** allow the **pelvis to roll and tilt away** from the body as the tailbone presses down to the floor. The **lower back** contracts and **arches** gently in response. The **chin is pulled down** towards the chest.

(the space between your hands expands as you move)

Movement 1 Finding Centre continued

3] As you **exhale** let the back slowly soften bringing you to the starting, or neutral, position (the place of non-effort).

Pause before repeating the movement.

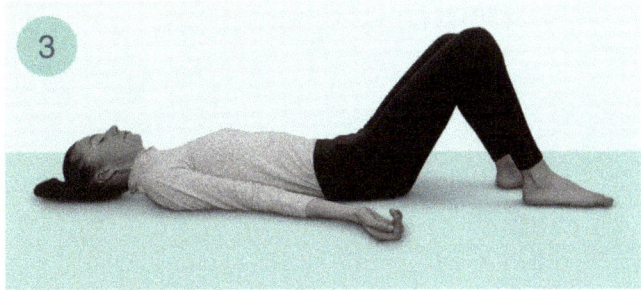

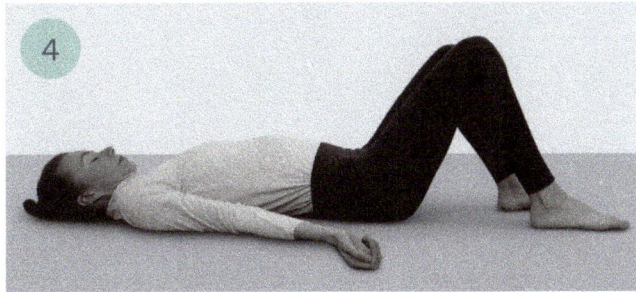

4] **Inhale**, roll the pelvis away, the lower back gently arches. The neck is long, **chin down** towards the chest.

Gently **press the shoulders** back into the floor to connect the upper body.

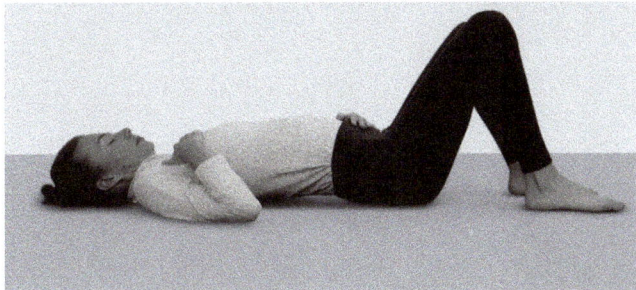

Notice how the front of the torso is expanded and open, the back contracted.

Slowly soften the contraction to release and return to centre.

Explore this 3 - 5 times.

Remember this can start as a small movement, growing incrementally with each repetition

Part 2 (Flatten) Contracting the front, soft relaxed back.

In your own practice you may choose to begin moving from either Part 1 or 2. You may find one aspect is easier to connect with, or more challenging.

5] Lie on your back with the **knees bent**, feet flat on the floor, arms rest alongside the body.

[Optional] Place one **hand over the lower** belly and one on the **upper chest** for feedback as you move.

This time take a breath in at rest. On the exhale start to move into the pattern.

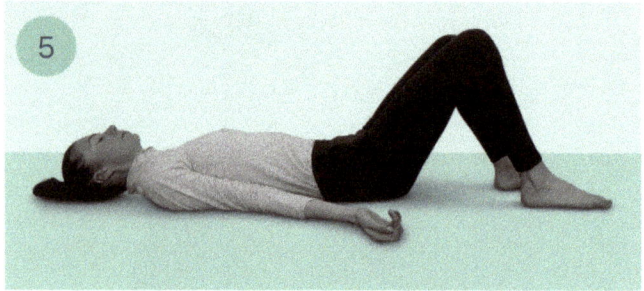

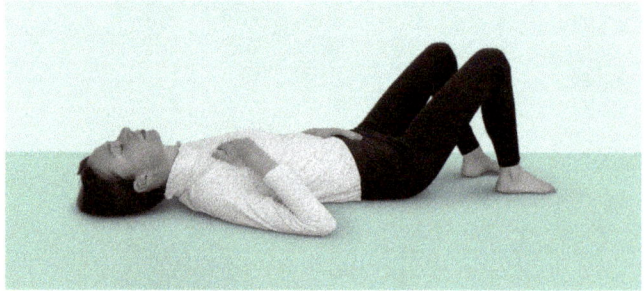

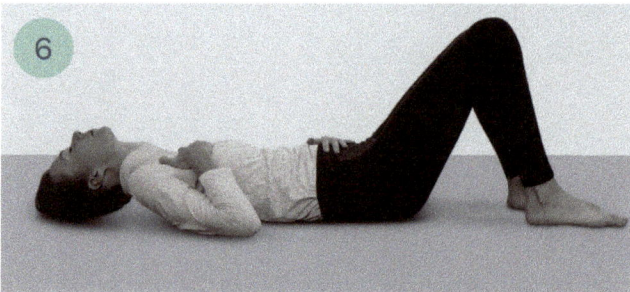

6] As you **exhale**, **contract and shorten the front** of the torso. The **pelvis tilts towards** the body as the abdomen contracts.

(the space between your hands decreases)

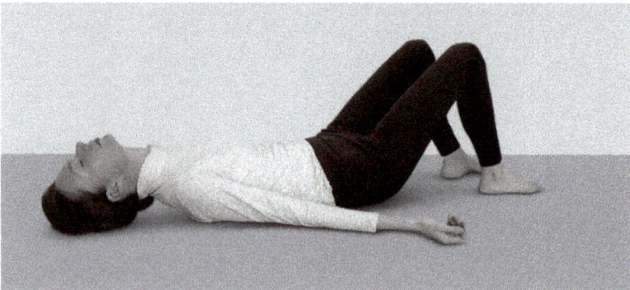

The **sternum sinks** and the shoulders round inwards in response.

Let the chin tip up away from the body (rolling on the back of the head).

7] To release, as you **inhale** slowly **lengthen out** of the contraction returning to the starting position.

Pause before repeating the movement.

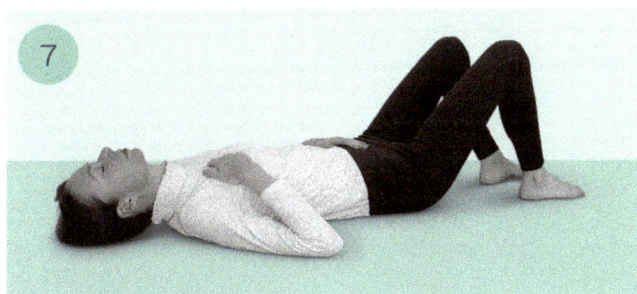

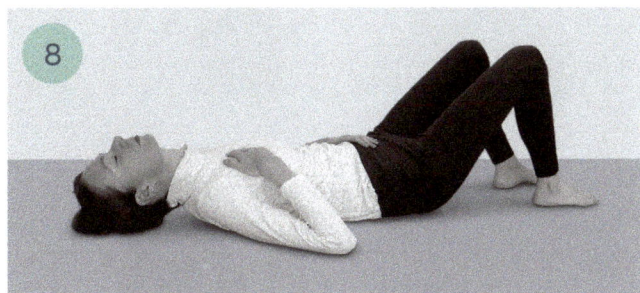

8] To repeat, use the **exhale** to move into the flatten. *The abdomen contracts to bring your hands closer together.*

Check the sternum (the upper chest and ribs) is also sinking down to join the pattern.

The **head tips back** away from the body. If it doesn't naturally want to follow, tip the chin up to encourage.

Slowly soften the contraction to release and return to centre. *Explore this 3 - 5 times.*

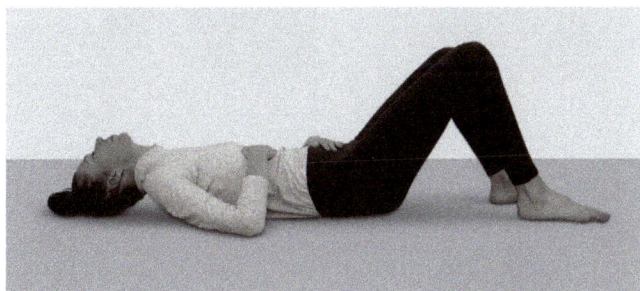

This is a movement and contraction from the front - check the buttocks are relaxed and not lifting or clenching!

Part 3 (Arch and Flatten)

Having explored each half you can then combine this into a slow wave-like movement.

You can coordinate the movement with long breaths flowing between arching and flattening or you can rest and reset in the centre.

9] Begin in the centre. **Inhale** and expand the lower belly like a balloon. **Move into the arch**, roll the pelvis to tilt away from the body, lower back arches. Shoulders press back into the floor. Neck is long, chin down towards the chest.

Slowly release on the exhale.

Either pause in neutral and reset with the breath, or continuing the exhale sinking down, into the flatten.

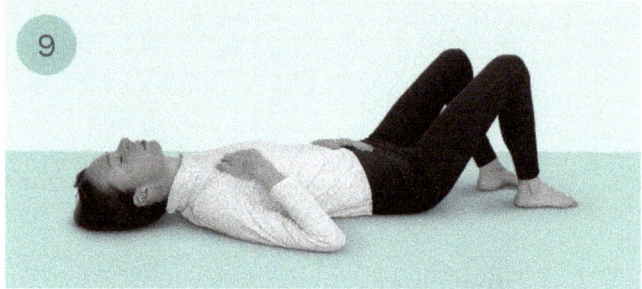

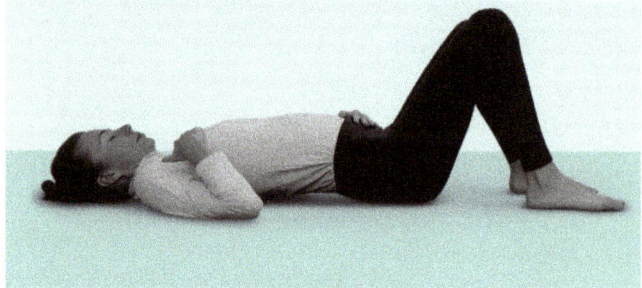

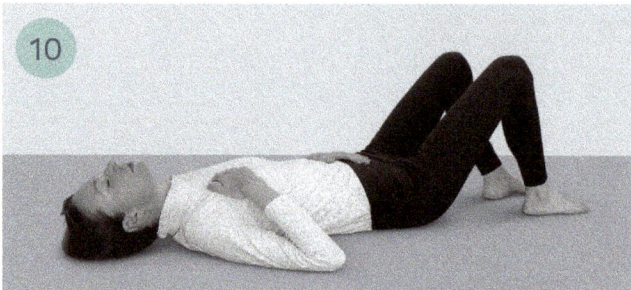

10] As you move through the centre use the **exhale** to **contract and shorten the front** of the torso.

The pelvis tilts towards the body as the abdomen contracts. *The back is relaxed and flat.*

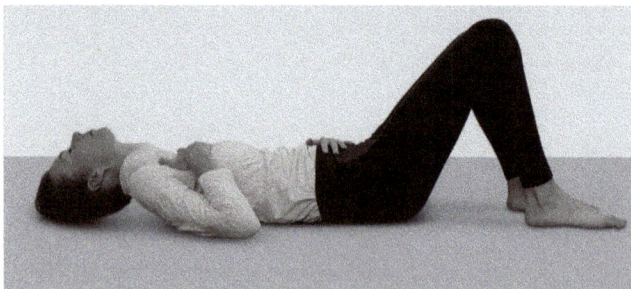

The **sternum sinks** and the shoulders round.

The **chin tips up** away from the body (rolling on the back of the head).

Movement 1 Finding Centre continued

11] Start to slowly release as you **inhale** and **lengthen out** of the front contraction.

Either pause in the centre and reset or continue moving into the arch as one long inhale.

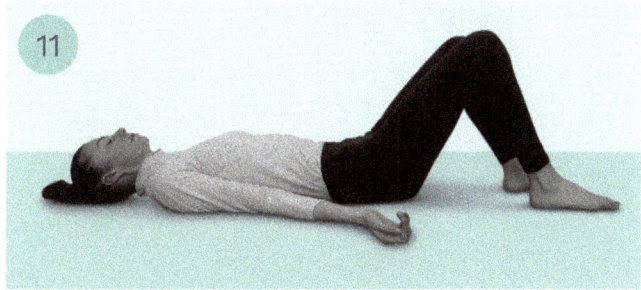

After exploring this wave-like movement a few times take an integrating pause in the centre.
Notice any shifts or changes...a flatter lower back? Space for the breath to flow in the front?

Notice as you move if you are being drawn more to one side. Do you roll straight down the centre-line or is there a pull or tilt to the left or right side as you arch or flatten? We will look at this next

Movement 2
Rebalancing Centre

When you notice that the first movement of Arch and Flatten is tilting or pulling you more to one side then including a recalibration early on can be helpful.

This movement follows the principles of the first movement but using diagonals (left hip-right shoulder, right hip-left shoulder).

First we do more of what the brain and body already wants to do, so if you noticed you were being pulled more to the left side of the pelvis, then start with this as your focus diagonal before moving to the other side.

1] Lie on your back with the **knees bent**, feet planted, arms rest alongside the body.

[Optional] You may like to place the **hands on the diagonal** for feedback (upper quadrant and the opposite lower).

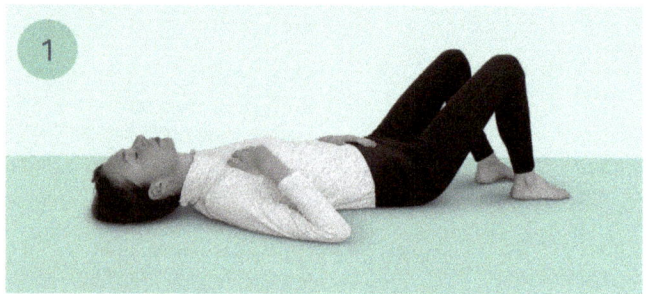

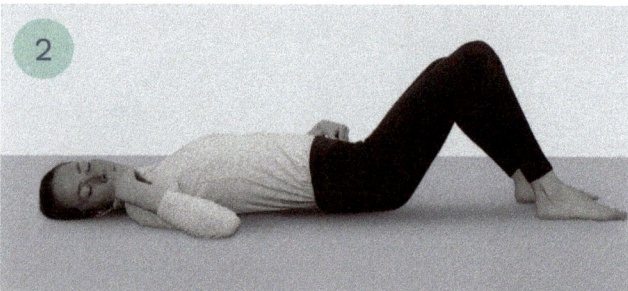

2] Diagonal Arch
As you **inhale** start to gently **arch over onto the left side** of the pelvis.

Press the opposite **right shoulder back** into the floor. The chin comes down towards the right collarbone.

You are making a gentle diagonal arch.

Notice the weight shift between the left and right sides of the pelvis

Use the exhale to release and return to the centre.

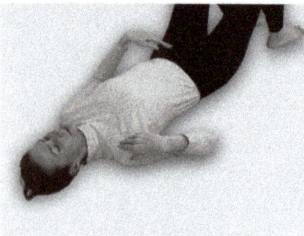

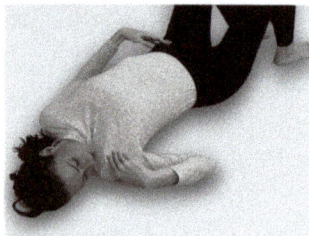

Explore this movement a few times before moving to the other diagonal (right hip, left shoulder).
You can also move from exploring the Arch to then exploring the diagonal Flatten before changing sides.

3] Diagonal Flatten

On an **exhale** move into the **flatten on the diagonal**, contracting and shortening across the torso – the **left hip** and **right shoulder** will slightly **curl towards** each other. The chin/head tips back away from the body.

You are making a gentle diagonal flatten.

Slowly release out, using the inhale to return to centre.

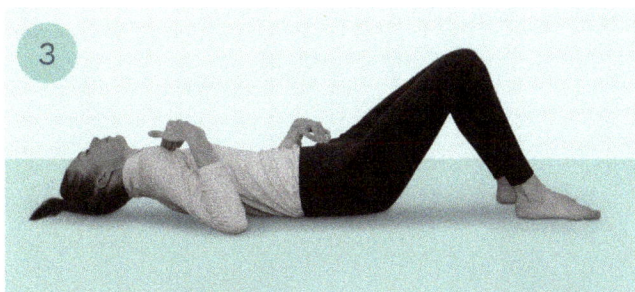

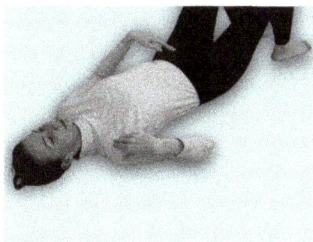

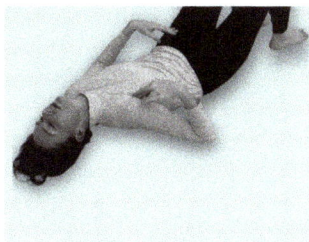

Repeat this movement a few times before exploring the other diagonal (right hip, left shoulder) shortening and contracting through the front.

4] Optional: Putting it together

Once you have a sense of each diagonal pattern you may like to explore moving between the arch and the flatten of each diagonal, using the breath to help coordinate the wave-like movement.

For example: inhale and arch over to the right side of the pelvis, at the same time pressing the left shoulder gently back into the floor. The chin will come towards the left collarbone. Slowly release out. On the exhale, contract into the flatten on the same diagonal, it's as if the right hip/pelvis and the left shoulder can curl towards each other. The chin tips up and away from the body.

You may notice that one diagonal is easier to sense or connect

What has changed?
Return to the original Movement 1 of Arch and Flatten and notice if you are now moving in a straighter line down the centre, or with less pull towards one side. What has changed for you?

PART TWO

Front of the body

front

Supporting the front of the body

Rounded shoulders, forward head, tech neck

The movements for supporting the front of the body focus on front flexion and taking us into forward, curling, rounding patterns.

This helps to mimic posture patterns like rounded shoulders, where the front is contracting and drawing the shoulders inwards. In response to this there is often a forward head and neck position. What's being called 'tech neck' today as it reflects our use and habituation with modern technology.

In this somatic pattern, for the lower part of the body there may be a tucking of the pelvis, where the contraction and rounding through the front pulls the pelvis and torso into a flexed, curved position.

It was once a posture traditionally associated with older age and frailty – the picture of the stooping, bent, or hunchback person. But now, in our modern technology world, we are adopting this at any age as we curl over devices for hours at a time.

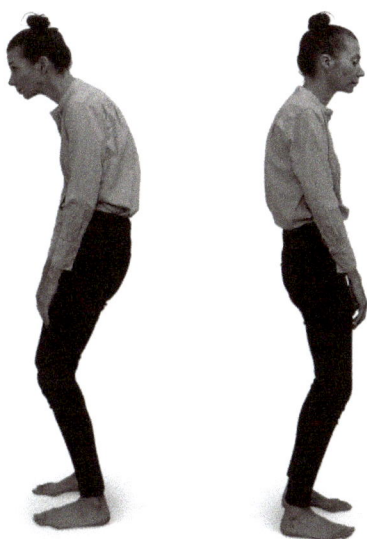

If we are not elderly then it is not surprising to hear a corrective call to 'stop slouching' or 'stand up straight,' 'pull your shoulders back.' Which is what we then try to do. We try to create the 'desired' outcome, to force the alternative, the opposite. We may even have to recruit a lot of other muscles in the process, like arching the back.

But as soon as we stop trying – or become consciously unconscious again – those shoulders won't naturally stay back. The brain and body are operating with a different understanding, a different (autopilot) program, a different habit and muscle memory.

To create a pattern change we have to engage both the body and the brain in order to consciously disrupt. We have to teach and release where it might be holding on (sensory-motor education), so our brain and body can sense, feel, learn and coordinate a different possibility.

It is finding and remembering the ease of potential instead of exerting effort.

This is what the somatic movements for the front of the body help to do.

A protective response to life

Curling inwards for safety, protection and security is an innate instinct shared across much of our animal kingdom.

As humans this physical response, rounding to withdraw or become small, also makes sense when we consider the front of the body is home to a lot of important (vital) organs. Being upright and forward facing is being open and vulnerable. We are exposed.

The action of curling and rounding through the front is also familiar, comforting even. It is the foetal position. And it links to our early startle response when we're an infant. A reflexive pattern of moving into flexion that we will look at more in the developmental section next. As adults, we still retain aspects of this automatic and protective response.

Just as movement repetition and physical actions can influence our postural habituation, we can also consider the energetic qualities within patterns.

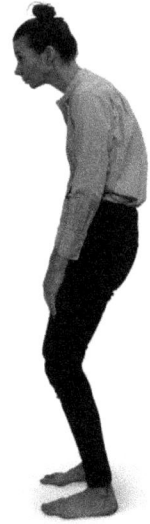

Our thoughts, feelings and emotional responses also impact our posture.

For the front of the body, moving in to flexion may mirror the feeling or need to withdraw, to stop, to protect, to move (even collapse) inwards. When we think about postures that go with expressions like: 'to protect our heart' (closed) vs 'opening our heart' (expansion) then we get very different physical, postural, energetic representations. This is part of being a human, considering all the parts.

There is a place for mind-body movement education, alongside other therapies, to help change long-held patterns or prevent them becoming ingrained in the first place.

We can also see how having patterns of muscular contraction could become counter-productive to our overall function, particularly if it creates restrictions. A chest that is sunken and a tight abdomen may impact our ability to breathe deeply and fully, for the diaphragm to move. Whereas having a relaxed centre supports the organs of digestion.
Somatic movements support our function.

It is helpful to know that we have the movement tools to be able to offset and gently reset patterns of muscular holding and contraction that can arise through the front of the body.

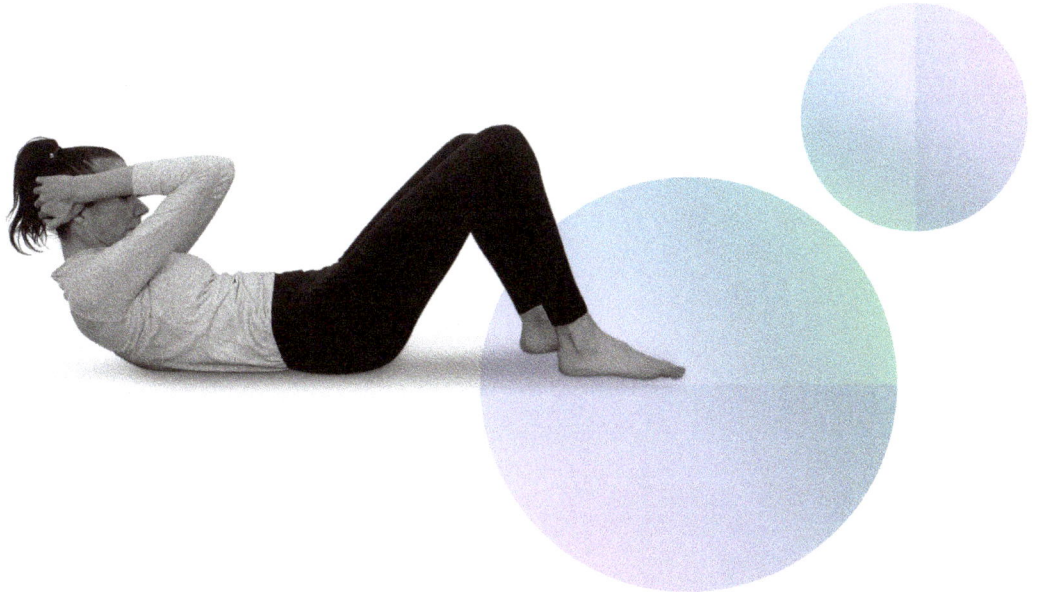

Developmental perspective

Our early startle response

When we consider flexion and curling through the front, it is where and how we all begin. From the time in the womb to the early months of being cuddled, carried and fed. It is the feeling of safety, security, nurturing, bonding and connection.

We even use it in our adult language when we talk about adopting the foetal position or just wanting to curl up. We generally have a sense of what this means or looks like, and what it feels like. And when we really hug someone we embrace front-to-front.

As a newborn it takes time to uncurl, to elongate and develop into upright beings.

It is an adjustment getting used to the front of the body opening up.

In the previous developmental section we looked at how the front of the body relates to the concept of 'centre' which also means feeling at home, or 'centred' in oneself. Working with the movements for the front of the body continues to build and strengthen this. We are also revisiting aspects of the early startle response, or moro reflex, which is an involuntary reaction in newborns.

The startle reflex is a specific and automatic response that can occur when an infant is startled by a loud noise, a sudden movement or feeling of falling.

When this fires, it triggers a physical and nervous system reaction. A cascade of internal and external activity. The arms and legs suddenly extend, the back arches and then everything curls inwards, and crying will often start.

It is interesting to consider that with this response there can be conditioning of our nervous system that is starting very early on. Everyday (and loving) acts such as picking up and putting down a baby, can depending on the method, inadvertently trigger this reaction. Which is why learning handling methods that support sensory-motor development can be helpful.

While the actual reflex becomes integrated over the early months, as adults we still retain aspects of this protective impulse that sees us round and withdraw in, when startled.

If you think about getting a fright, someone jumping out and saying 'boo,' then we have an automatic reaction and contraction occurring through the front. It is designed to protect us.

Just as we need the ability to move into patterns when life demands, we also need to be able to move out (fully) when it is safe to do so.

The movements ahead, while very beneficial for our postural habits and holding patterns are also beneficial for our nervous system.

To feel safe and at home, centred in ourself.

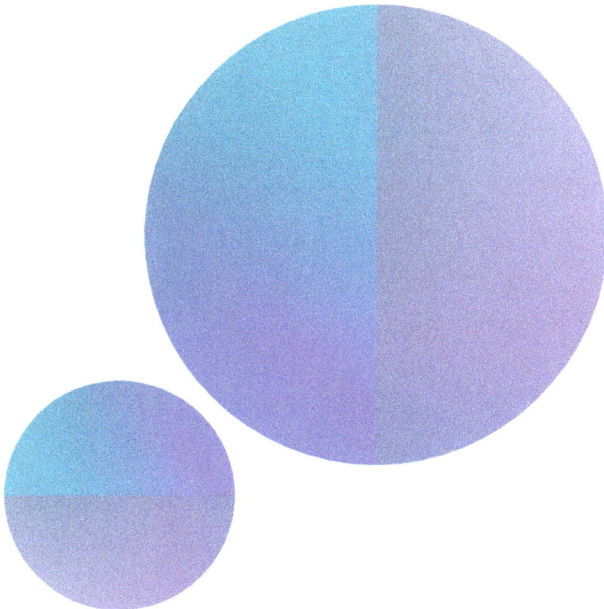

Movement 3
Arch and Curl

This movement builds on the first movement, taking the front flexion, the curling and rounding further into the upper part of the body.

Remember this is not a 'sit-up' or about using core strength. The lifting of the upper part of the body comes through the contraction of the front, the deepening into flexion.

We also have a front-back relationship and coordination occurring, as for the front to contract we need a back that can respond to the movement. The yin and the yang. This is a movement that, like so many of our somatic movements, we can grow incrementally, with each repetition. Starting small at first.

1] Lie on your back with the knees bent, feet planted. Interlace the fingers and clasp the hands beneath the head. Elbows rest on the floor. *If support is needed for one or both shoulders, place a rolled-up towel under the upper arms.*

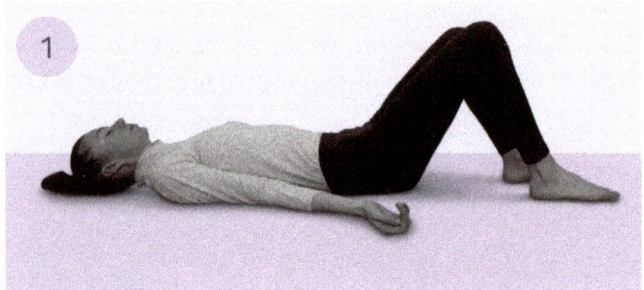

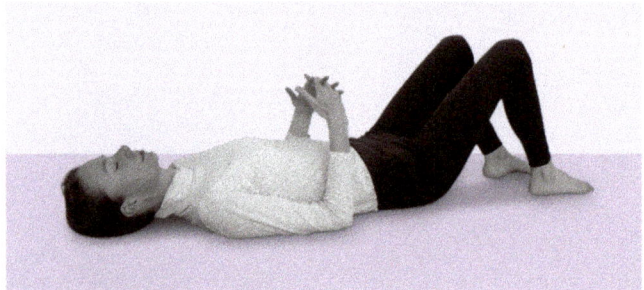

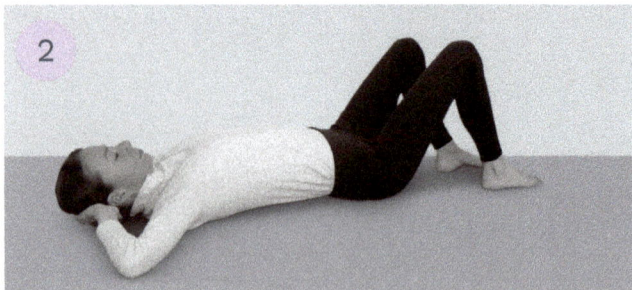

2] As you inhale and move into the arch, pelvis tilts away, gently press the elbows back.

Chin comes down towards the chest.

Movement 3 Arch and Curl   continued

3a] As you **exhale** and move through the centre (either pause here for a breath or) continue **into the flatten**, contracting through the front and flattening out the lower back.

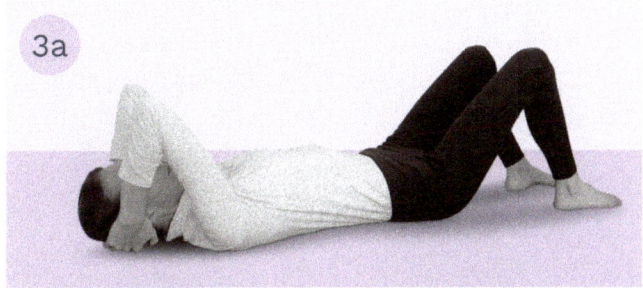
3a

3b] At the same time curl the arms around the ears and allow the **contraction** through the front of the torso to lift the head and upper part of the body. The **elbows** are pointing towards the knees/thighs.

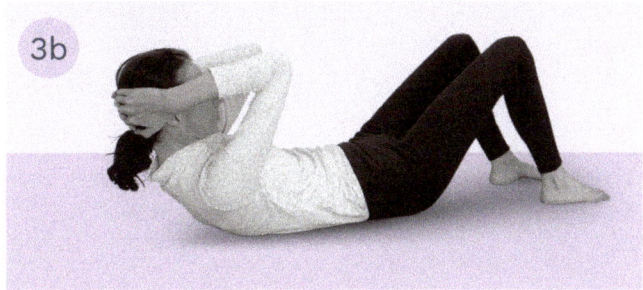
3b

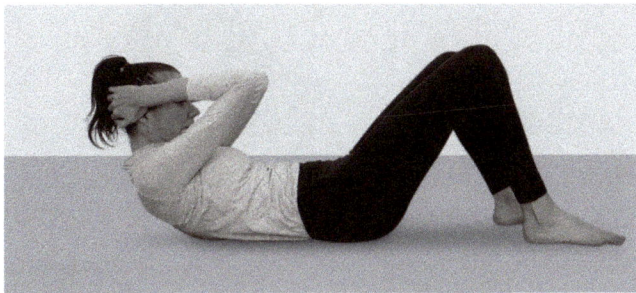

4] Use as **many breaths** as you need to slowly release out and **return** to the starting position. Completely relax before repeating.

Explore this 3 - 5 times.

If you notice shaking when you reach the top of the movement then just ease back slightly.

Movement 4
Flower

This movement continues the theme of supporting the front of the body. It builds on the earlier movements to create a full body pattern for the front.

In clinical somatics this movement is called the 'flower' as the motion is likened to the opening and closing of a flower bud.

It is re-creating the movement pattern, the flexion and rounding of the startle or withdrawal response, as well as the posture and habituations of modern technology – this is a great movement to do if you find yourself hunched over a computer, desk, device or driving a lot.

It is the 'rounded shoulders, forward head, tech/text neck' offset.

It can also feel soothing for the nervous system in times of stress or anxiety. It is a gentle reminder that allows the chest and shoulders to be naturally relaxed and open, creating space for the breath to flow.

1] Lie on your back with the knees bent, feet planted, arms extended alongside the body.

Notice and sense your shoulders before moving. Is one side sitting differently?

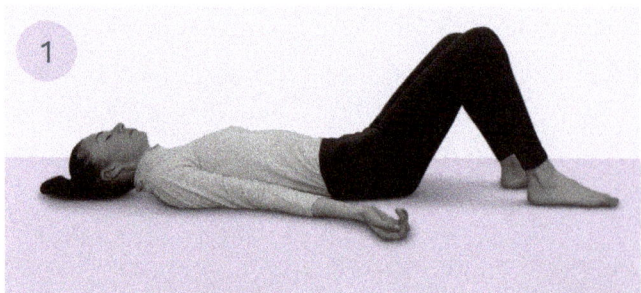

[Arm motion reference] Both arms will be moving together at the same time.

To spiral open, both shoulders press back into the floor the palm of the hands and arms roll open.

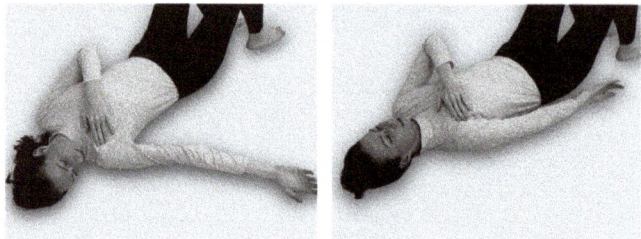

To spiral the arms inwards the shoulders round in (shoulder blades glide away from the spine) and the arms roll as the backs of the hands face towards the thighs/body.

The hands/fingertips stay lightly connected to the floor as the arms roll. No lifting the hands up off the ground!

Movement 4 Flower

continued

2] Inhale at rest. On the **exhale move into the flatten**, contracting through the front of the torso, sinking the sternum, **head/chin tilts back** away from the body. **Shoulders round, arms roll in,** backs of the hands face towards the thighs.

Moving within your comfort range.

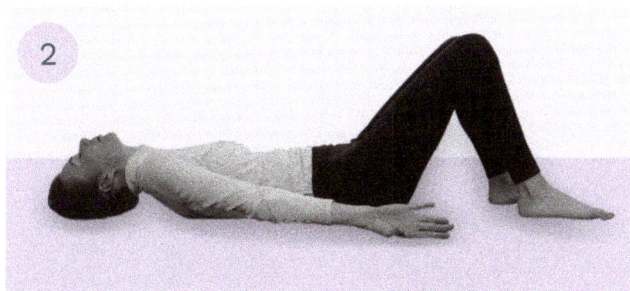

3] To release slowly soften out, return back to the centre. Pause and take a few resting breaths.

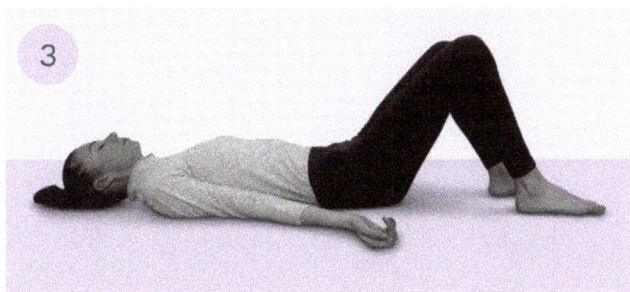

4] **Optional: Inhale and Arch** opening the front first.
While the focus is on the front flexion and rounding movement, we can also include the back of the body as part of this pattern.

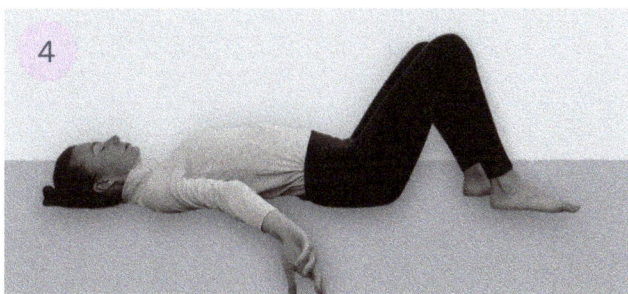

4] **Inhale** moving into the arch, pelvis tilts away, chin down towards the chest, **shoulders press back**, arms spiral open, palms of the hand open. *Remember not to go into stretch. These can be small movements to start with.*

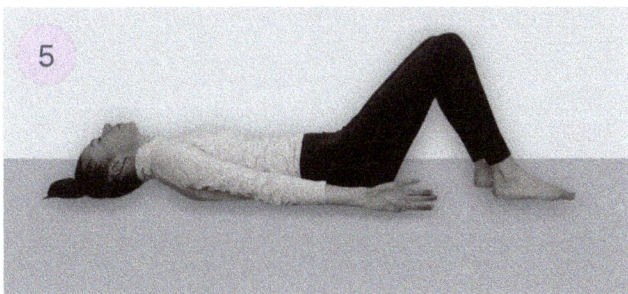

5] **Exhale** moving back through the centre, either pause and reset the breath or continue into the **flatten**, rounding the shoulders and spiralling the arms inwards. Check the **head/chin tilts back**, away from the body. Slowly release out.

Movement 4 Flower

continued

6] Optional: bringing the legs into the pattern

6] As you inhale and move into the pattern (pelvis tilts away, lower back gently arches, chin comes down, shoulders press back, arms spiral open) let the knees open a little wider apart. Use the exhale to reverse out, softening the back.

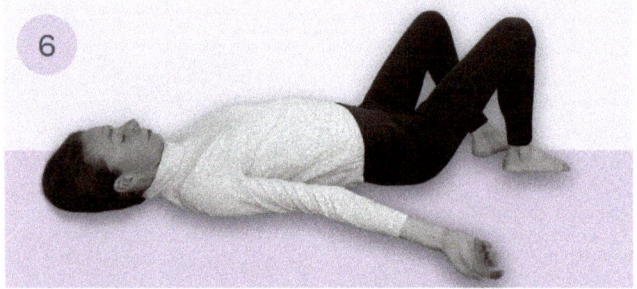

7] As you exhale and move into the flatten (sink the front, arms and shoulders roll in, head tilts back) let the knees come towards each other. You can gently squeeze/press the knees together.

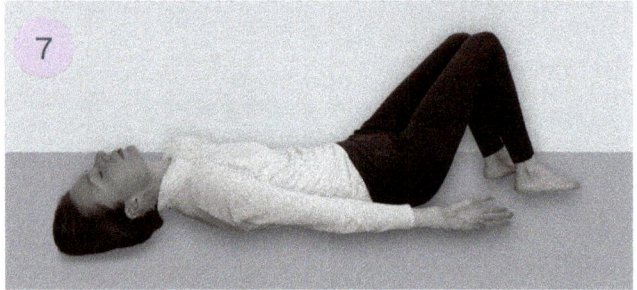

Here we have our 'flower,' opening and closing.

Explore this movement 3-5 times

Notice and sense any changes at the end. How do the shoulders feel? Is there more contact with the floor, or openness through the front?

What if there are jumps, skips or shaking in the movement?

As you move into or out of a pattern there can sometimes be jumpy, jerky or shaky parts to a movement.

If there is shaking as you contract into a pattern, like the deep flexion of Arch and Curl or the Flower, then we may be working a little too hard and creating more tension than is needed. Try easing back a bit.

As you release out of movements you may notice there can be jerky places or jumps, like the movement is skipping parts. If it was an elevator then we've just bypassed a few floors on the way down!

This is the idea of SMA (Sensory Motor Amnesia). The jumps or skips are highlighting where the brain doesn't have a clear or controlled sense in that part of the movement, and or muscle(s).

Sometimes it's not the range of movement that's the issue, but whether we are in control of it!

If you notice this jumpy aspect, then pause and go back into the pattern or movement, take your time to slowly, slowly release out, allowing the brain to notice all the parts. You may find the jumps become less, or a smoother connection and motion forms. Our aim is to be like a string of chewing gum – all parts connected.

Slowing down helps.

The slower you go, the more the brain and body can sense, feel and notice. This is where the learning, the education, is taking place. The unconscious becomes conscious - that which is needed for habit change.

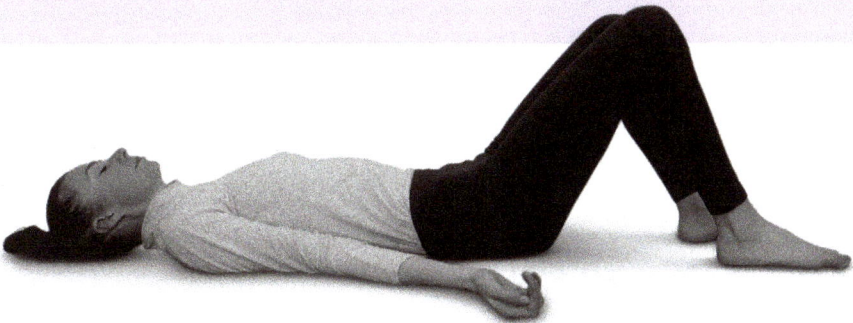

Are standing desks the answer?

When sitting was equated as the new smoking the boom in standing desks became the natural response. From a somatic postural perspective this was interesting, as I see just as many people holding patterns of muscular imbalance when standing! (and if you did the photo exercise you may have noticed your own unique patterns)

When we add concentration to a task we often become unconscious in other areas. If we're using our brain power on a computer task we may become unaware of how we are sitting or standing. Those old autopilot programs 'help us' out so we can direct energy elsewhere.

While the health advantages for standing over sitting certainly exist, it is still beneficial to bring awareness to our posture habits and patterns however we are using our body – particularly when it involves sustained periods of time.

Just as movements can be helpful to offset a pattern, like rounded shoulders from curling over a device, they can also set us up to operate from ease, like before we start working at a standing desk and holding ourselves upright.

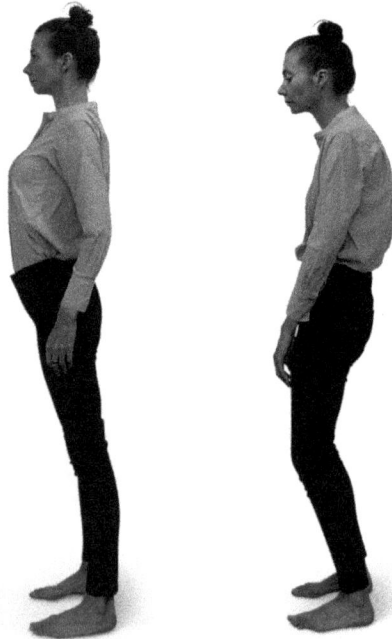

PART THREE

Back of the body

Back

Supporting the back of the body

Upright and forward motion

The movements for supporting the back of the body focus on extension and the patterns of being upright.

The muscles of the back play an important role in bringing us up into standing, keeping us upright as well as moving us into forward motion.

It is a unique part of our two-legged humanness.

In order to ready us for this action, the posterior extensor muscles of the back contract. It is the energy of 'go go go' – of being 'on' – and visually it can also look like this. Our posture might reflect someone standing ready to attention. The shoulders are back, the back is arched and it may seem like we're almost leaning or pitching forwards, we're that ready to spring into action.

But if these back extensor muscles are constantly held in contraction, like we're always on and ready (just in case) then it wouldn't be surprising to hear complaints of a tight, sore or tired back.

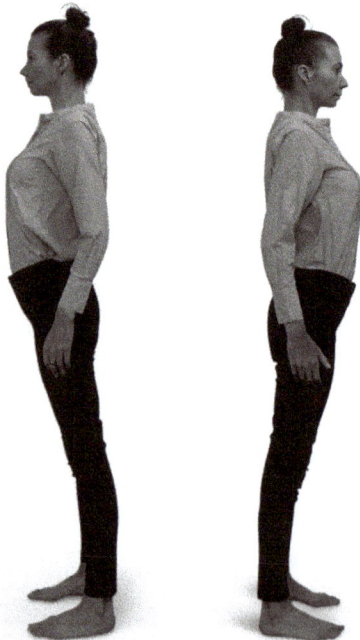

Imagine the feeling of lying down at night, or trying to relax after a busy day but with those back muscles still holding on.

It can be quite a reflective posture of the world we live in. The 24/7 doing, achieving, being busy and always on. The hustle. As well as the perceived value that may be ascribed to this. Like when someone asks, 'how are you?' and the reply is 'so busy' and that is seen as a good thing.

In the same way, there can be a view that this is a more desirable posture to have – an acceptable or positive pattern. Visually, it is the opposite of being rounded and withdrawn. The energetics are very different.

But we can also consider that patterns and posture may be presenting differently in different people. Just as fear, worry and anxiety is more likely to move us into contraction and withdrawal through the front, fear can also drive us to keep moving and striving forward. We can become addicted to 'busy' and conditioned to always being 'on.' To out-run ourselves and use the adrenaline of the back of the body.

If we're so busy doing (motor) then we don't have to stop and perhaps have to feel (sensory).

Here it is important to emphasise that individually, somatic patterns are neutral. One isn't good or bad, better or worse. **We need all of them.**

We need to be able to move into and out of them as we respond to life.

It is only when a pattern becomes habituated, and is contributing to muscular imbalances leading to pain, discomfort or restriction that we might start to realise we're no longer in neutral territory. For the back of the body, this may impact on our structure, like our spine.

This is why we have our somatic movements for the back of the body. To bring awareness and control. To help offset and come out of patterns so it is less likely to become a habit.

Back pain from chronic muscle tightness isn't something to strive for. And if you find yourself thinking you are too busy for somatic movements then you definitely need to be doing them!

A sway back is not a sexy back

One of the common patterns appearing for the back of the body is the idea of a 'sway back.' This describes the forward sway of the lower back, or the lordotic curve of the lumbar spine area. If you were to feel the muscles either side of the spine here then they are usually very tight. With this contraction and shortening of the lower back area comes the sway, sending the abdomen forward in the front.

It is a curve that the fashion world accentuates and high heels exaggerate. But it can affect anyone with a back!

The irony of addressing a tight lower back - softening those contracted lower back muscles - is that it reduces the sway that is sending the tummy forward. Clients, both male and female, have commented on the appearance of a flatter tummy as a positive bonus to their somatic movement practice. It is also a lot more effective than trying to pull, or 'suck the tummy in' using the front when the back is already working hard to send it forwards!

It is difficult to go anywhere when you have your foot on the brake and the accelerator at the same time.

From my own experience, and that yoga class, I discovered that what I thought was a weak core was, from a somatic perspective, a tight lower back. When I learned to release and coordinate the front and back together, then I found neutral. I was able to access and engage the muscles of the front. I had and was in, control.

Remember that to change a long-held unconscious pattern we need an educational disrupter.

This is what somatic movements gently, yet powerfully do. It is a reminder of a different possibility. And that true strength is supple strength, rather than a ridged holding.

When working with the movements of the back it is important to listen to your body and to work gently, to work somatically. You can build up to movements incrementally. There is no end goal or award for achieving here. There is only what is right for you, and what is right, right now.

The relationship and interplay between the front and back of the body is also like a dance. To be able to move into extension through the back then it helps for the front to be released. Before exploring movements for the back individually it is recommended to include Movement 1. This helps to coordinate the front and back moving together and address areas of potential tightness or holding that could be happening in the torso centre.

Developmental perspective

Becoming upright

While the first few months for an infant centres around the front of the body, the next big phase will be the developing back of the body.

It is a step-by-step journey as muscles develop and connections form that will see a progression into becoming upright. From the early prone or tummy-time position, to moving to all fours, cross-crawling and eventually into a freestanding and two-legged explorer.

This idea of 'becoming upright' is both about the physical aspect and our inner sense.

What it is to stand in ourselves, to hold ourselves upright, and to stand on our own two feet. So that when life inevitably knocks us around we have the ability to find our centre, return upright and move forward again.

The back of the body is also about support and feeling supported. Our 'backing' in life.

We use these ideas already in our language with expressions like 'I've got your back' or 'that's an upstanding person – their character is upright.'

When it comes to then working with adults and somatic movements I like to consider the two movement roles, or aspects for the back:

There is being upright itself. What it is to stand effortlessly in ourselves. To find connection, balance and symmetry through the back.

Then the second part is taking this uprightness into forward motion. The cross pattern of walking and how different quadrants coordinate and connect through the back.

The movements ahead explore this.

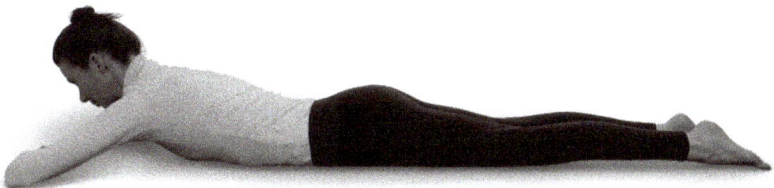

Movement 5
Backlift 1

Bringing awareness and coordination to the muscles of the back. Exploring connection, symmetry and balance through the back of the body.

Remember to start small, move slowly and always work within your comfort range.

If you are exploring these movements out of sequence or individually then set this up with the first movement (arch and flatten).

After exploring back extension work then it can be beneficial to return to some front flexion afterwards. Movement 3 Arch and Curl can be a helpful counter-balance to this.

1] Lie on your front with the legs extended, **folding the arms** in front so that you can rest the forehead on your hands.

Prepare to move by imaging the crown of the head and neck is being pulled long.

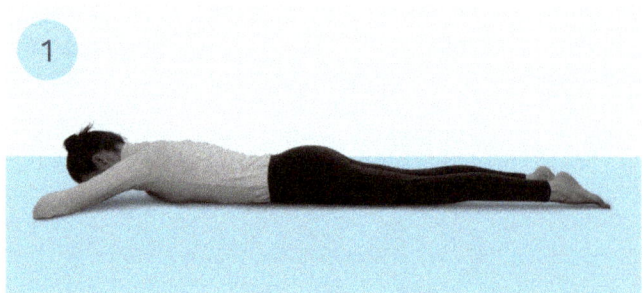

2] **Inhale** and start to **lift** the head/neck/upper body a little.
This lifting movement comes from the muscles of the back.

Slowly release back down and rest in the starting position.

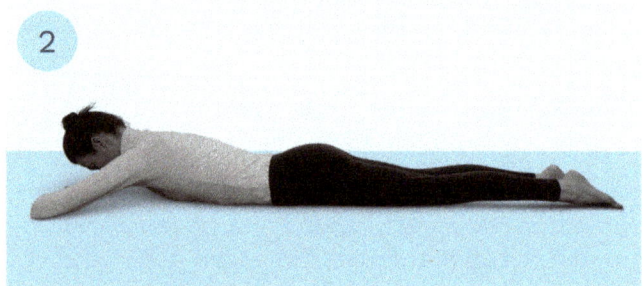

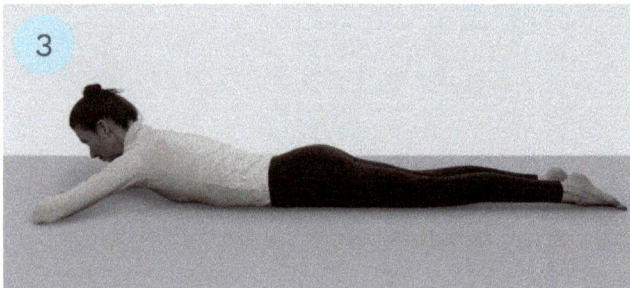

3] When you are ready, repeat this movement.

Noticing with each repetition you may come slightly higher.

Explore this 3-5 times. Rest and relax the back between repetitions.

Movement 5 Backlift 1

Option: adding the legs
Rest the upper body as you explore the lower connection with the legs.

4] Rest the upper body. Start with the **right leg**, as you **inhale** let the right leg reach away from the body and **lift off the floor** a little.

Notice the connection into the lower back and contraction of the buttock.

Exhale and slowly lower.

Take a moment of pause as you switch everything off (relax the glutes/buttocks).

Explore this 3 times.

Then repeat this for the **left leg**.

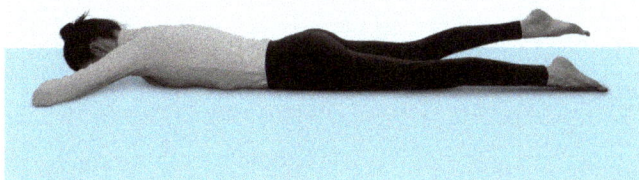

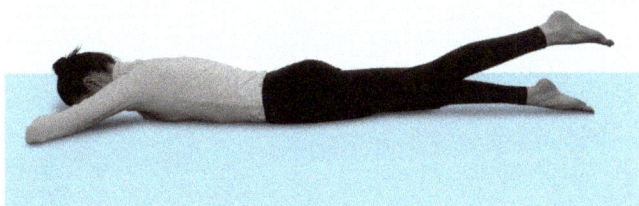

Remember these can be small movements

Option: combine upper and lower together

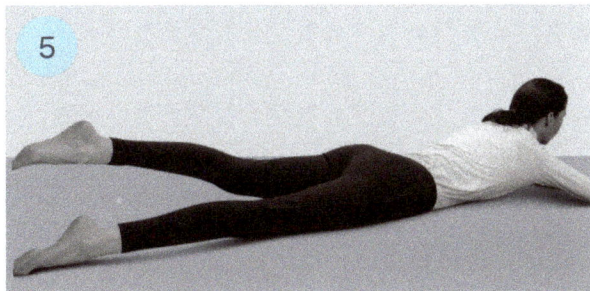

5] Inhale and **lift** the upper body and the (left) leg.

Slowly and with control **lower** the upper and lower body together. **Relax** completely when you arrive.

Explore this again with the other (right) leg lifting.

Movement 6

Backlift 2

Bringing awareness and coordination to the muscles of the back. Exploring cross-patterns through the back of the body that support forward motion.

Remember to start small, move slowly and always work within your comfort range.

If you are exploring these movements out of sequence or individually then set this up with the first movement (arch and flatten).

This movement can be broken down into parts and then put together. Let's explore this:

Upper body

1] Lie on your front with your **head turned** to face your left.

Bend you left arm, so the elbow is out from the body, fingers pointing towards the nose/face, palm of the hand and arm resting on the floor.

Your other arm (right) is at rest alongside the body.

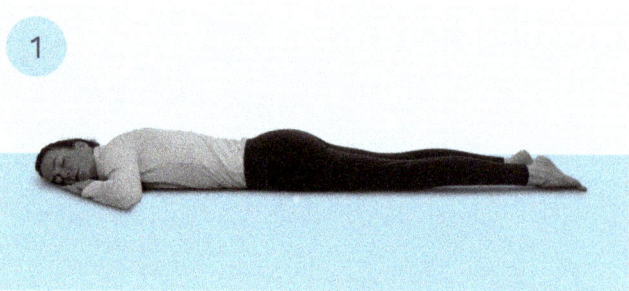

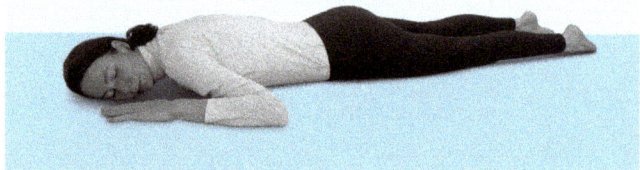

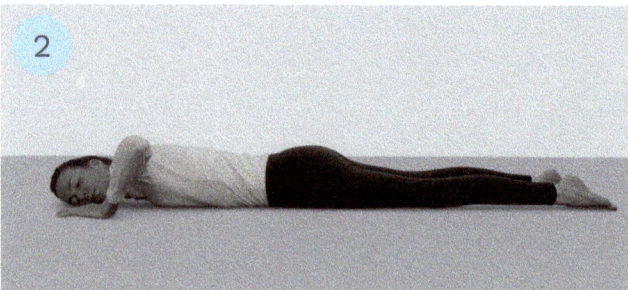

2] Inhale and slowly float just the **elbow up** (palm stays flat on the floor), exhale as you slowly lower down (notice any jumpy, jerky, shaky parts)

Explore this 3 times.

Movement 6

3] Inhale and use the muscles of the back to **lift just the head** a little, exhale to lower down. Rest then repeat.

Explore this 3 times.

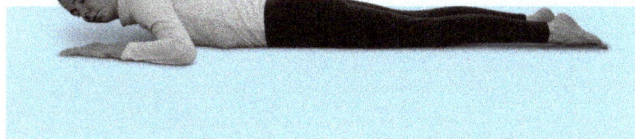

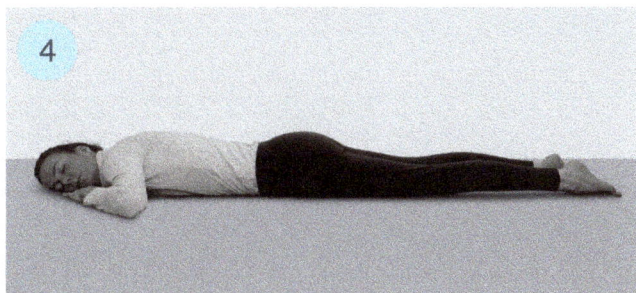

4] Next, slip the fingers underneath the cheek or have the fingertips against the side of the face. *They will stay connected as you move.*

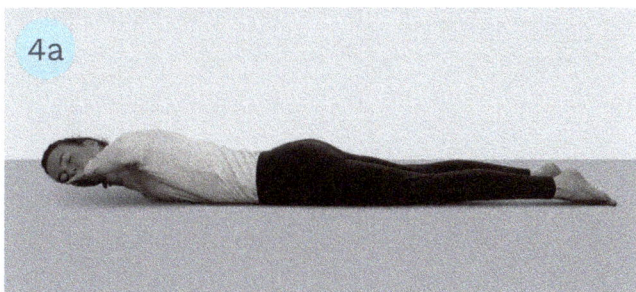

4a] In this part the **elbow, hand and head all lift together**. Use the inhale to help you lift, exhale as you slowly lower down. *Explore this 3 times.*
Lift within your comfort range. This can be a small movement to start with, just off the floor.

As you feel comfortable to grow the movement notice how the elbow can lift towards the ceiling, as if you could look over your shoulder.

Notice the connection into the shoulder and upper back.

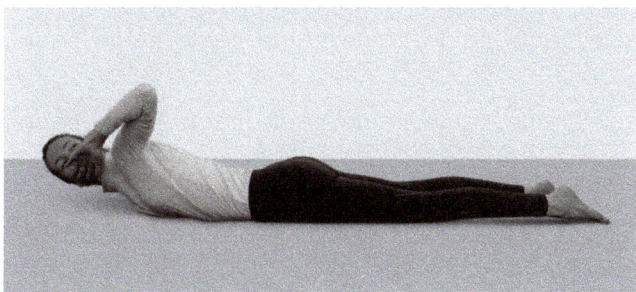

(You may start to sense the opposite leg wanting to lift)

Movement 6 Backlift 2

continued

Lower body

5] Rest the upper body as you bring your awareness to the opposite side leg (right leg). Inhale and **lift the leg** a little off the floor. Exhale and lower.

Explore this 3 times.

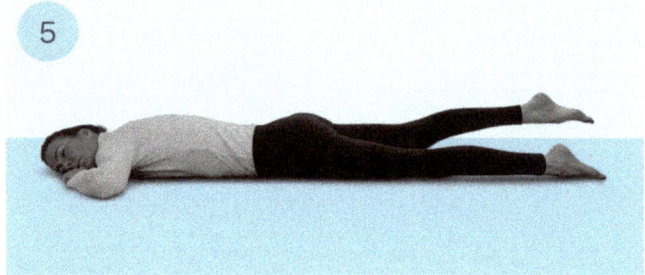

Putting it together *Visualise, start small.*

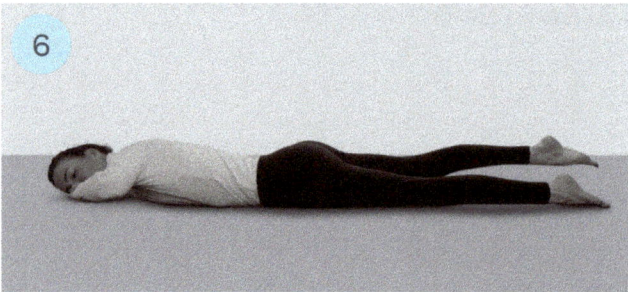

6] Putting it all together: Inhale into the belly, lift the elbow, hand and head and opposite leg.

To release back down, slowly lower with control.

Relax and then repeat.

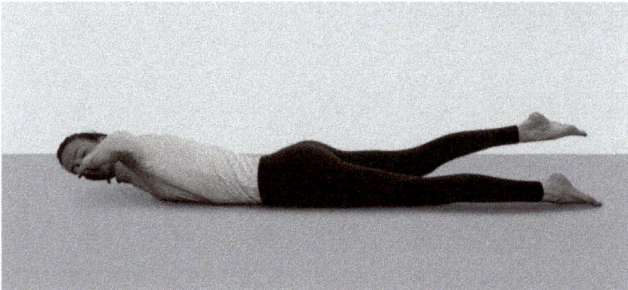

Explore this 3 times then move to the other side.

Visualising this movement first can be helpful as it is coordinating a little bit of movement in a lot of places.

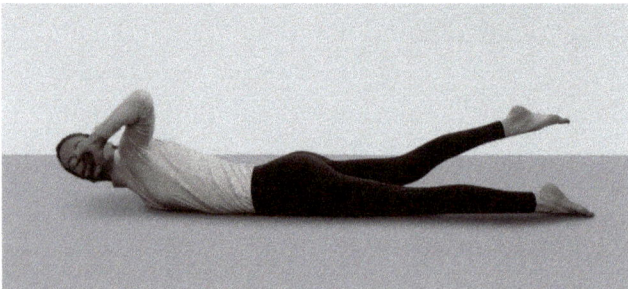

Start small and grow the movement incrementally.

Moving only within your comfort range.

Movement 6 Backlift 2

Switch sides

7] Follow the same steps for the other side.

Explore:
2] Right elbow lifts x 3
3] Head lift x 3
4] Head, hand, arm lift x 3

5] Opposite (left) leg lifts and lowers x 3

Then:
6] Put together x 3

Notice the diagonal connection between the upper right quadrant and the lower left through the back.

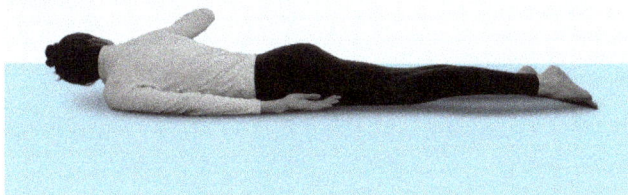

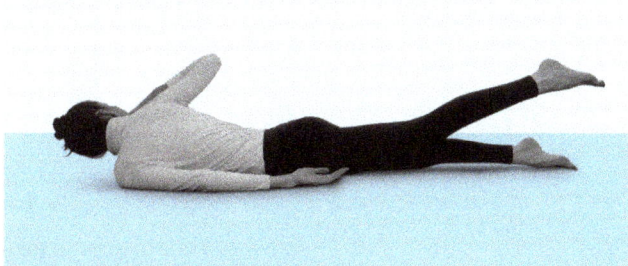

After exploring back extension movements it can be beneficial to follow with some front flexion. The Diagonal Arch and Curl (Movement 7) is a great counter-balance

Feeling it in the lower back?
Back extension work can feel strong! If it feels like the lower back needs a break, bring the head to rest in the centre, bend the knees and slowly windscreen-wipe the legs from side to side (just a small movement). Follow then with front flexion, like Arch and Curl to counter-balance.

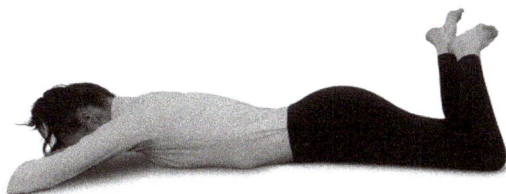

Movement 6a
Backlift 2 Variations

The full, original movement of the Backlift can be a little strong when first learning or if there are known, existing issues.

There can be different ways of approaching or adapting somatic movements that still give the benefit and intention of the original movement. The following variations offered encourage the cross-lateral connection of the muscles of the back, and that which supports our upright movement patterns of walking and forward-motion.

Upper exploration
This exploration builds on the first movement for the back (Movement 5) engaging the muscles of the back, lifting and lowering the upper quadrants.

1] Lie on your front with your **head turned** to face your left.

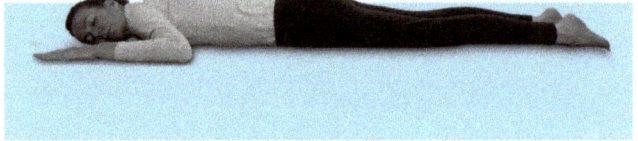

Rest the arms on the floor at right **angles** from the body – a bit like a sphinx.

Inhale and **lift the head**, neck, upper body (using the muscles of the back),

Slowly turn the head into the centre-line (so you are looking down at the floor).

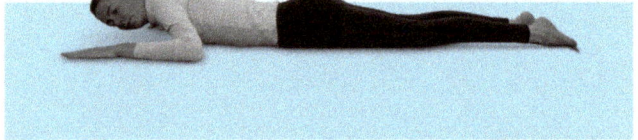

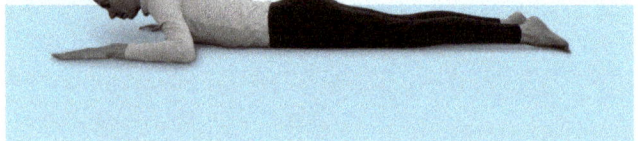

Movement 6a Backlift 2 Variations

Continue to turn the head and neck to look to the other side and slowly lower down on this side as you exhale.

Pause and rest here. Then repeat the movement lifting from this side.

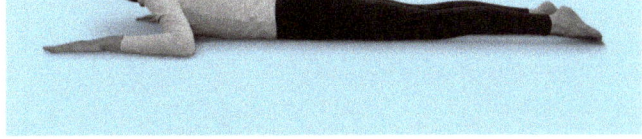

Noticing the connection and movement of the head, neck, shoulders and back as you lift and lower.

Explore this movement a few times.

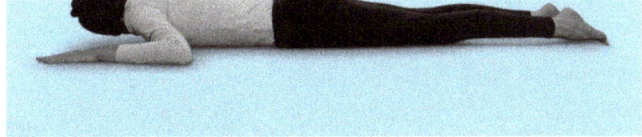

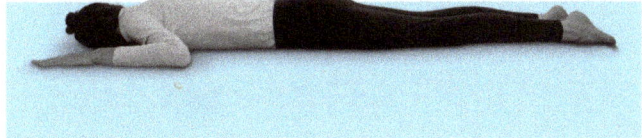

Modified Backlift 2

This movement is a modified version of Backlift 2. Visualising this movement first can be helpful as it is coordinating a little bit of movement in a lot of places.

1] Lie on your front with your **head turned** to face your **left**. The left will be the focus lift side for the upper body.

The arms can either be positioned at right angles (see previous movement) or set up like the Backlift 2 (p68) where the non-working arm (right) is at rest alongside the body

Explore inhaling and lifting the head, as if you could glance over the left shoulder. Then lower back down.

The elbow can either stay in contact with the floor or it may lift as the shoulder blade glides on the diagonal. *Work within your comfort range.*

You may notice the opposite (right) leg wanting to join the pattern as you lift.

The next time you lift the upper part of the body, allow the opposite leg to also lift. *Here is the diagonal connection through the back.*

Slowly and with control lower both the upper and lower together.

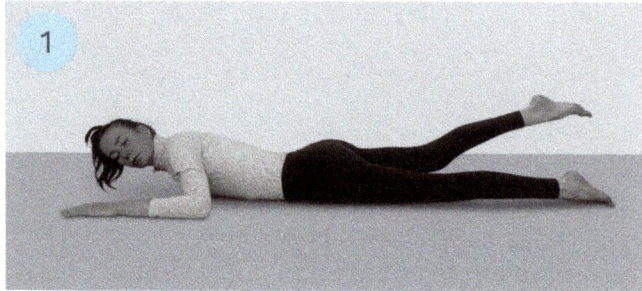

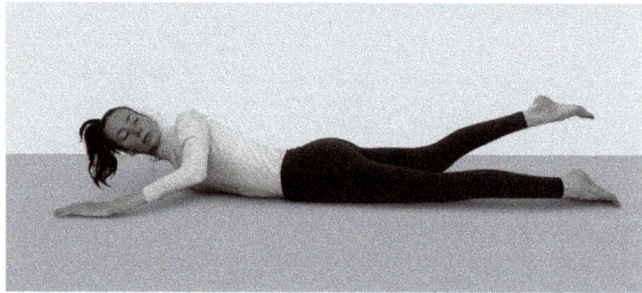

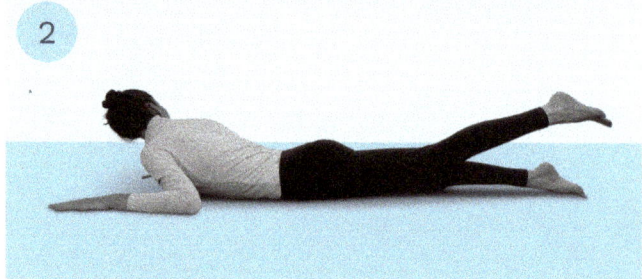

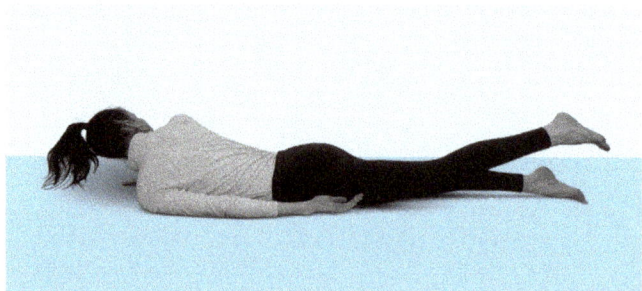

2] Explore this a few times before moving to the other side (right upper, left leg). *Repeat x 3.*

Movement 7
Diagonal Arch and Curl

This movement is similar to the Backlift 2 but with a front focus.

It continues working with the diagonal quadrants, like we did for the back, but through the front of the body, and into flexion.

It is a helpful movement to do following Movement 6, revisiting front flexion after back extension.

The movement follows the principles of Movement 3 (Arch and Curl) but working diagonally.

1] Lie on your back with the knees bent, feet planted.

Place your **right hand under your head**. Draw the **left knee in** towards the body and allow the left hand to rest on the thigh or clasp the knee.

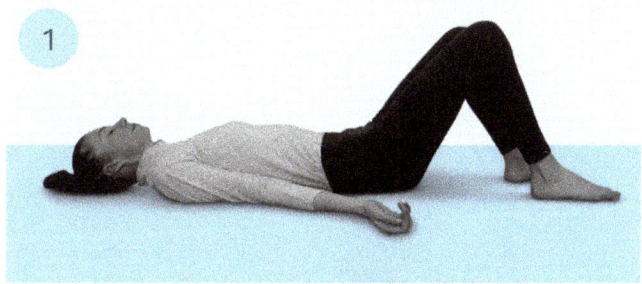

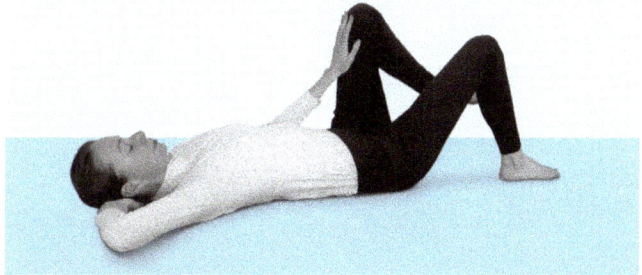

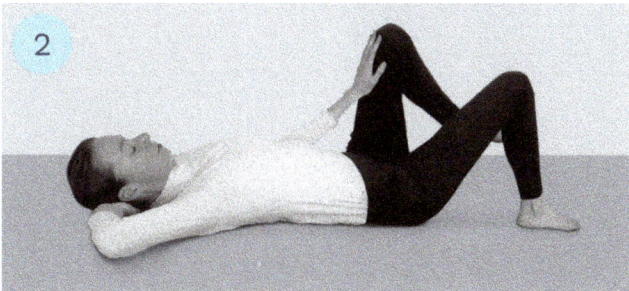

2] **Inhale**, move into a gentle arch as the pelvis tilts away from the body. Chin is towards the chest.

Press the **right elbow back** towards the floor (if comfortable).

You can let the knee/leg float away, the hand can slide along the thigh.

3] **Exhale** and let the back sink down, moving into the flatten, contracting the front of body.

The knee will come closer towards the body.

The **right elbow curls** around the ear and the muscles of the front contracting helps to lift the head and curl the elbow in the direction **towards the left knee**.

Breathe as you need.

To release slowly lower back down, floating the elbow to rest and knee back.

You can rest your foot down in between repetitions if you need.

Repeat two more times before moving to the other side. (left hand behind the head, bend right knee)

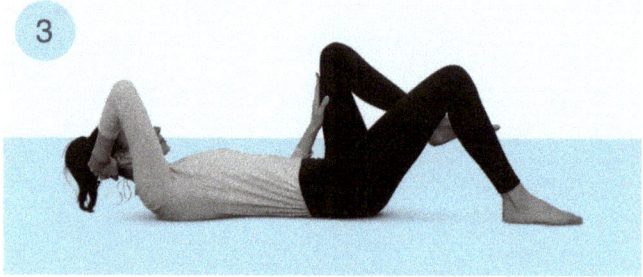

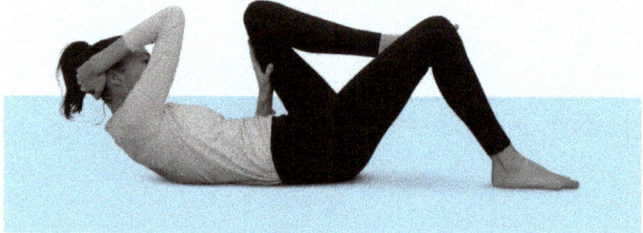

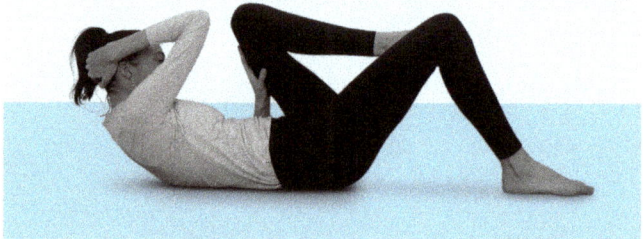

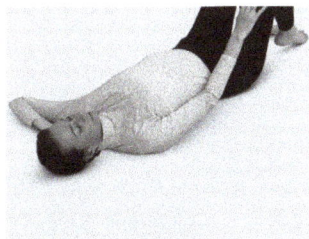

4] Prepare to move the **other side**, place your **left hand under your head**. Draw the **right knee in** towards the body, right hand rests on the thigh or clasps the knee. **Inhale**, move into a gentle arch to set the movement up, **left elbow presses back.**

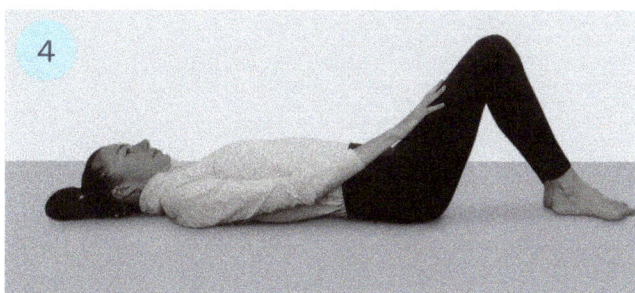

5] **Exhale** sink down into the flatten, **left elbow wraps** around the ear and the muscles of the front contracting helps to lift the head and curl the elbow in the direction **towards the right knee**.

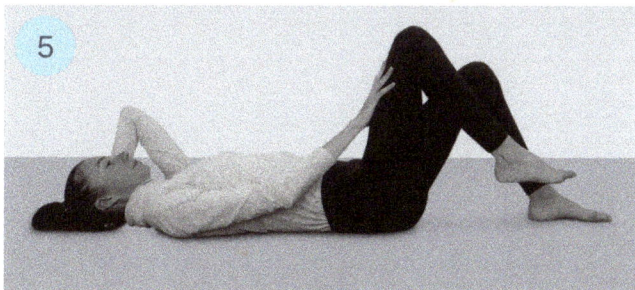

Breathe as you need.

To release slowly lower back down, floating the elbow to rest and knee back.

You can rest your foot down in between repetitions if you need.

Explore 3 times each side.

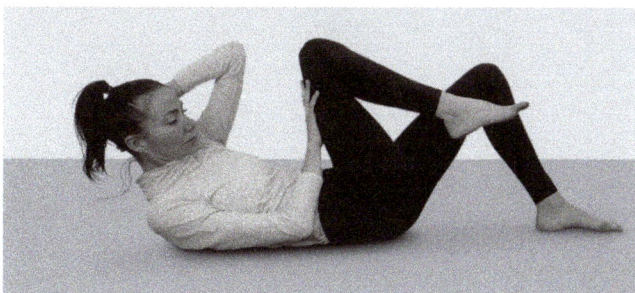

PART FOUR

Sides of the body

sides

Supporting the sides of the body

The movements for supporting the sides of the body focus on the side waist area. Our side-to-side movement and connection.

This has a lengthening and shortening dynamic, a bit like an accordion opening and closing. As well as connecting the upper and lower, the lateral aspects of the body through our sides and waist.

When there's an imbalance through the muscles of the side waist area it can contribute to other functional imbalances in our posture as compensatory patterns occur to help keep us upright and our horizon line level.

The irony of this adjustment which helps to keep us going straight is that the rest of us can become a little wonky. A zig-zag of sorts in order to balance the imbalances.

Visually it might appear as uneven posture. In standing, you might notice that there are different curves or gaps on either side of the waist between where the arms fall. Or that clothing may bunch and gather differently in places. There might be a tilt of the head and neck. The shoulders can appear uneven or one arm looks to be longer than the other. In this case it is not that the actual arm lengths are different, but that it is occurring as

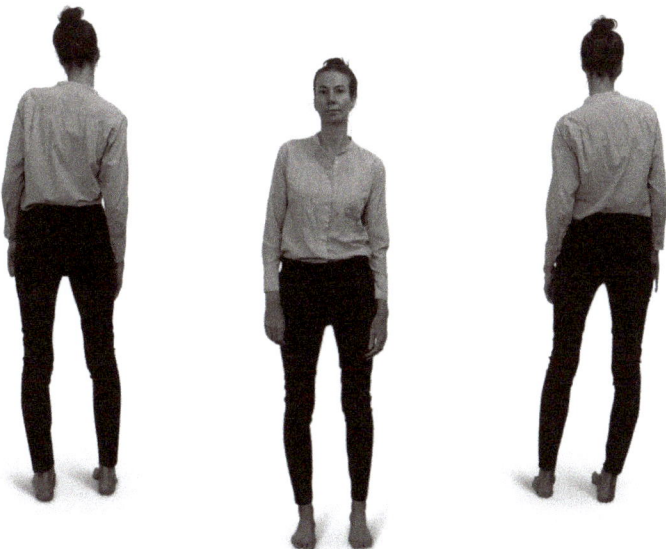

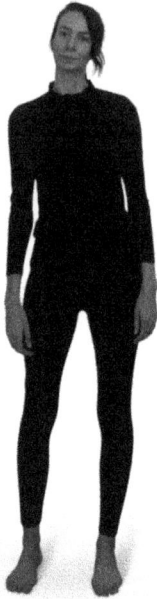

a result of a pattern of holding and contraction elsewhere. The same can be viewed with the legs and a tilt of the pelvis higher to one side.

When there is not a true limb length discrepancy it is more likely to be a postural response, like contraction through the waist that arises from a one-sided event or repetitive action to one side.

When there's been an accident, injury, surgery or sudden impact to one side, then the muscles of the waist curve and cringe as a response to help protect, guard and avoid pain or further damage.

If we take the example of a sprained ankle. In order to avoid pain and further damage we have to shift our weight off that foot and leg and modify how we move for a while. You can feel for yourself what happens when you shift your weight off one leg in standing – there's a big adjustment through the sides of the waist. To ensure that we don't topple over to one side, a righting response or compensatory patterns then occur to counter-balance us.

In time that ankle heals and we go back to regular activities. We might not even think about the injury any more.

We may have rehabbed the ankle, but not retrained the rest of us.

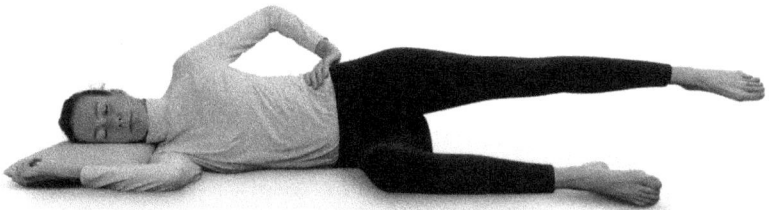

Unconsciously, we could still have a level of muscular holding and imbalance through our side waist or the various counter-balancing patterns. This might not cause any discomfort or issue straight away and so it continues to stay out of our awareness.

Years or decades may pass.

Until we notice some sort of new pain or discomfort or restriction creeping in. It might not be anywhere near the foot so we don't associate it with that old ankle injury. Sometimes clients even forget they had an injury (or which side it was even on). But the conditions, the subtle holding and habits could have been set in motion a long time ago.

Such a pattern can arise without something traumatic but simply our everyday habits in life. For example, carrying a bag over the same-side shoulder, picking up and carrying a small child on one hip, playing a sport or musical instrument that dominates to one side of the body.

It is our habits and adaptations, combined with time, that can become an uneven posture.

It is a bit like compound interest for the body but choosing which direction to go.

We can either unconsciously add to our existing patterns and habits, thereby strengthening and reinforcing them over time, or, we can start to add a somatic movement practice now and see the investment and return benefits over time.

Smart muscles, smart brain.

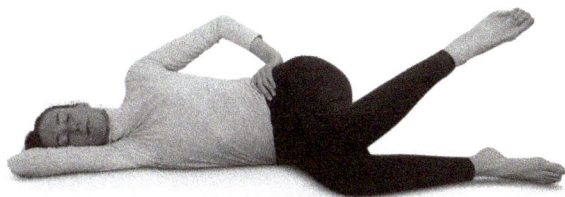

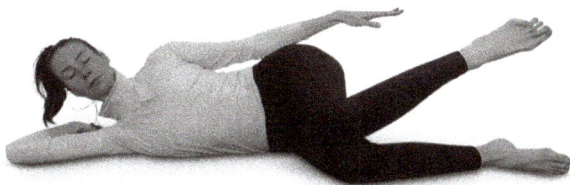

Underpants on at 80

While ageing itself may be inevitable, a decline into disease or disability isn't. The areas we do have some control over is empowering.

Whenever I don't feel like the motivation to practice (because, like you, I'm human, and winter mornings are cold!) then I think about 'underpants on at 80.'

Because if we are fortunate to live long lives, then I want to live it well and to move well, and I want that for others too. What it is to age with grace, independence, dignity.

It is also such a gift to start before you have pain, before there is an issue. We may still need the supports, advances and interventions of modern medicine. Joints may still need to be replaced, but we can also have movement tools to support us throughout life. To help us to keep doing the things we love to do for as long as possible.

The sides as a confusing place

My own experience in learning somatic movement was to discover that the sides can be a confusing place. Particularly when there has been accidents or injuries in the past.

Initially it felt tricky to sense and connect, to feel and coordinate.
Is there the ability to lengthen one side while shortening the other?
Is one side as smart as the other?

I felt anything but smart when it came to the sides!

Subtle shifts can also have flow on affects for our proprioception, as our sense of where we are is also adjusting. Straightening up a tilt of the head and neck can put us in a new reality that then feels a little wonky.

The sides of the body are also home to important life themes around rotation and flexibility, as well as supporting our balance and playing a key role in fall prevention. Maintaining and sustaining this is part of what keeps us youthful and curious. Let's see how this begins in development.

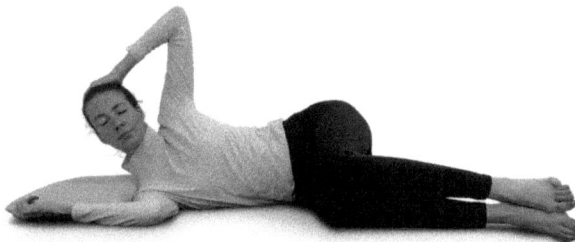

Developmental perspective

Rotation, curiosity, flexibility

For an infant the developing sides of the body sets up the themes of rotation, flexibility, curiosity and exploration ahead.

As before this, we are stuck. We are stationary creatures in the sense that where we are put down and placed is where we stay. We cannot move on our own yet. We have to develop this ability.

At around the fifth to sixth month we start to form the movement of being able to rotate from being on our back to turning over onto our tummy. Then a few months later comes the second part of turning, moving from our front to our back again. This is a fun skill to practice over and over again as now, we are rolling!

We are no longer limited to a fixed place or position. Rotation means our world and possibility is opening up.

The precondition for this movement of rotation is the ability to shorten and lengthen the sides of the body. To coordinate this.

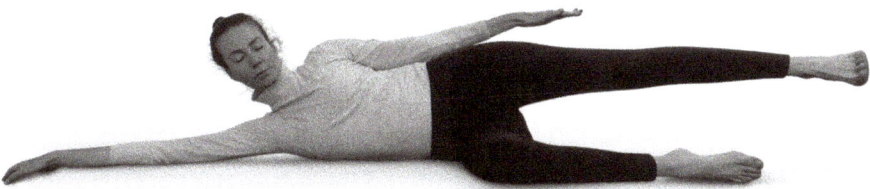

Sometimes babies will use hyper-extension (at any age) to arch the back and flip themselves over. It is a way of turning but it is not true rotation by engaging and developing the sides. It is more like flipping a banana than coordinating the lengthening and shortening of the waist. As care-givers, we can learn handling methods so that when moving and turning a baby it is also supporting the sensory-motor development of the sides to come.

There are some that might argue, 'well why does this even matter? If they get there, they get there.' Which is true, but these early skills have a flow on affect into later years and seemingly unrelated abilities. Such as when it comes to **stumbling and fall prevention** (which is important at any age) and the ability to catch our balance or use our arms to reach out to break a fall and protect our head. As well as to be able to pivot and change direction, to move around our axis, when we need.

All this starts from the early development of the sides of the body. Of learning to rotate and coordinate our waist, arms and legs.

Breaking a fall, or falling flat on your face

Some years ago a friend fell while on a holiday. They hit the ground face first and the dental work required was significant. Their partner had wondered why they hadn't put their arm out to break the fall, which can help protect the face and head. But they just had no instinct or muscle memory to do so and as a result toppled like a falling tree trunk.

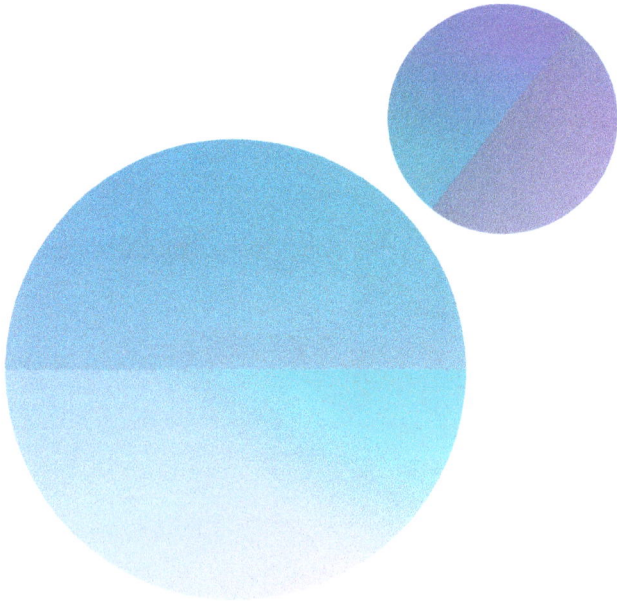

Last to develop, first to go

While the phases of early sensory-motor development are not occurring in isolation or separate to one another they are themes which we carry with us throughout life.

There is an idea that if we start to lose the ability of rotation, whether we're 30 years old or 70, then we've started ageing, a declining process that sees development go in reverse.

This is not just the physical but also the internal, the body and the mind, our flexibility in thinking and emotions. If rigidity creeps in there can be quite fixed ways of thinking or being, of set routines and fixed times for things like meals and activities. We can become resistant to change. Unbending, unyielding. It can happen at any age.

Finding ways to support the sides of the body, to maintain our rotation and flexibility, our supple strength, is so important, especially for ongoing balance and fall prevention as we get older.

Development in reverse

I've come to see the ageing process as being a lot like the phases of development but in reverse. As once we lose rotation and flexibility our world narrows. Where do we turn when we can't physically turn? Our path and our possibilities can become limited, fixed even. The fear and potential for falling grows as balance and motion changes.

Then if our back support weakens we become hunched, less upright, maybe reliant on a walking aid to help us shuffle forwards. We may become even less mobile or unable to move on our own accord. Fears which contract us inwards.

For some this may continue further into flexion, mirroring our early beginnings and dependence – requiring care, feeding, cleaning and reliant once again on others for survival.

While no one knows what's around the corner in life, it can help to know and prepare the smart muscles, smart brain way today.

We want to be able to bend like the willow, rather than break like the oak.

Movement 8
Gentle Waist Movement

This movement is a gentle way of addressing the sides while lying on your back. It is about bringing awareness, connection and coordination to the muscles of the waist.

Unlike other movements that require a firm surface beneath for feedback, this is a movement you can do in bed as the focus area is on the side waist area moving.

1] Lie on your back with your knees bent, feet flat on the floor. Arms rest alongside the body, or, you may like to place your hands on the hips to feel the movement.

Breathe as you need.

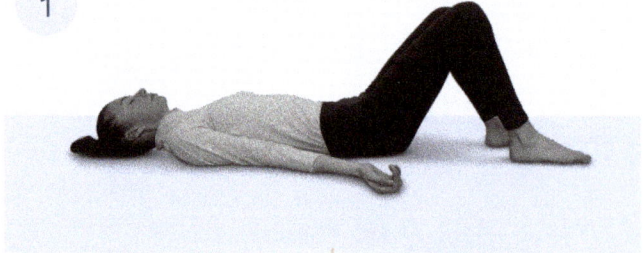

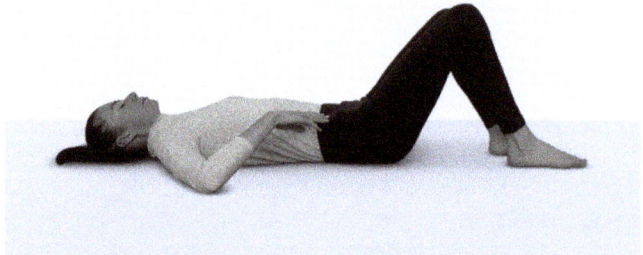

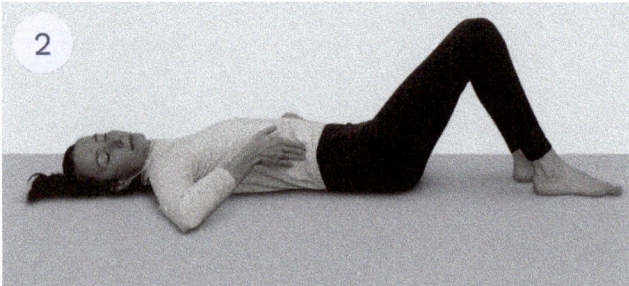

2] Begin with the right waist, slide the right hip up towards the right armpit, the muscles of the **right waist contract and shorten**, and the left waist will lengthen in response.

You can place a hand on the side waist area to feel and check that it is these muscles working, it will feel tight as you contract and shorten.

Movement 8 Gentle Waist Movement   continued

3] Release the waist to bring the pelvis level and the hips centre.

Explore this 3 times on the right side.

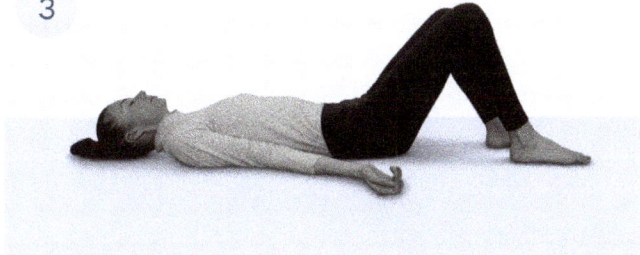

Option] Arm reach: The arms rest alongside the body. As you contract and shorten the right waist let the right arm slide slightly away from the body along the floor.
This is a subtle movement to bring in the upper side waist.

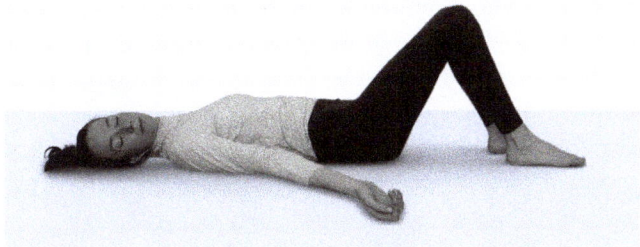

Remember the back stays flat and in contact with the floor, no arching up as you move.

4] After exploring the right side **move to the left** waist and repeat the movement on this side.

5] Once you have a sense of the movement you can **alternate moving side to side** – contracting the right, releasing to centre, contracting the left. Making 'c' shapes side-to-side. *Notice the steering wheel-like motion beneath your hands as the hips/pelvis move.*

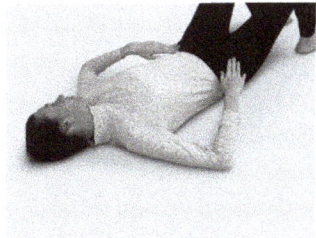

Notice as you make these 'C' shapes through the sides of the waist if the head wants to roll with the movement

Movement 9
Sidebend

The focus area in this movement is the muscles of the waist along with connecting and coordinating the sides of the body. Below are the steps for the classic or 'original' sidebend movement, followed by variations and alternatives for the arm and leg positions that you can explore.

As an exercise with a lot of moving parts, it is beneficial to first explore each and then put together to build the full movement.

1] Lie on your **side** with your legs at **right angles** to your waist.
It is as if you are sitting in a chair (sideways).

You may like to place some support under the head, like a folded towel.

Align the head, neck and back in a straight line.

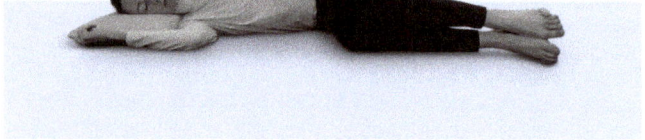

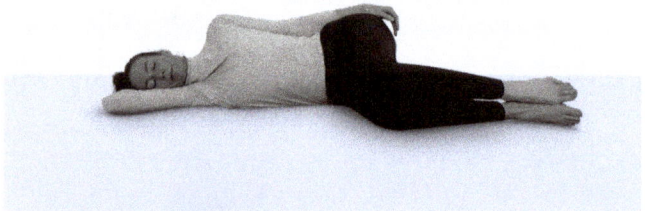

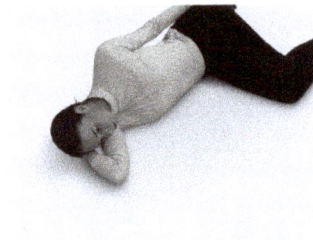

You can also use your underneath arm as a resting support for the head if it's comfortable. Either bend the elbow of the lower arm as pictured or have the arm extended long (see image 3.b, p91)

Movement 9 Sidebend <inline style="color">continued</inline>

2] Lower body: bring your hand to the topside waist so you can feel the contraction.

Inhale to the topside waist to set the movement up. **Exhale** and keeping the knees together **float the top foot** up a little, noticing how the **waist contracts** and shortens (as if your hip could slide up to your armpit).

Slowly lower the foot as you release and lengthen the waist muscles.

Explore this 3 times.

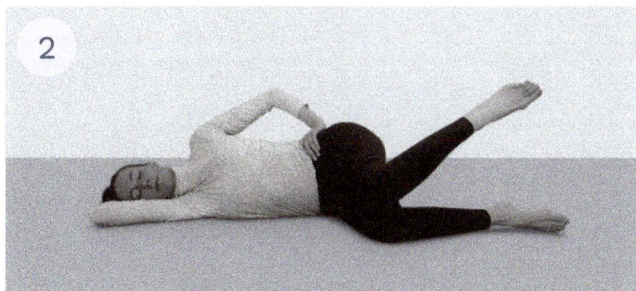

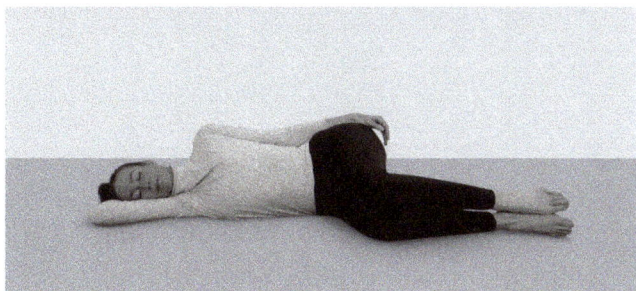

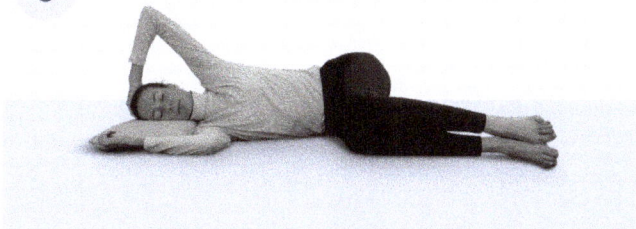

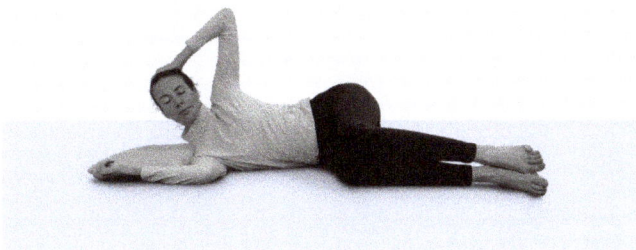

3] Upper body: next, place the arm over your head and gently clasp the top of the head.
Keep the elbow high.

(Or use an alternative arm position: 3a, 3b, p91)

Inhale to expand the top ribs, **exhale** and slowly **contract the side waist** in a straight line down towards the hip, **floating the head up**.

Slowly lower back down.

Explore this 3 times.

As you lift it can help to keep looking straight ahead to ensure you are moving from the sides and not twisting/ curling the neck forwards or back.

4] **Put together:** upper and lower movements.

Inhale to expand the topside waist (accordion is open). 4a] Exhale, contract the waist muscles, floating the top foot up, head lifts (accordion is closed).

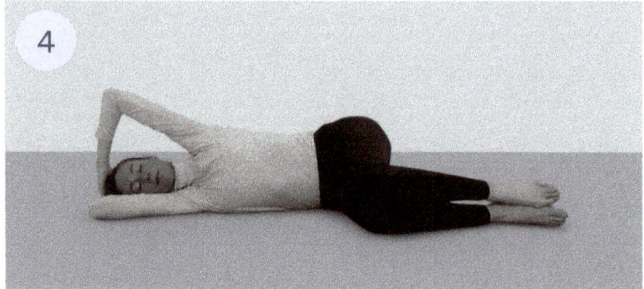

Slowly lower back down, releasing from the waist, seeing if the upper and lower body can land at the same time. Rest and relax.

5] Explore this 3 times then change to the other side.

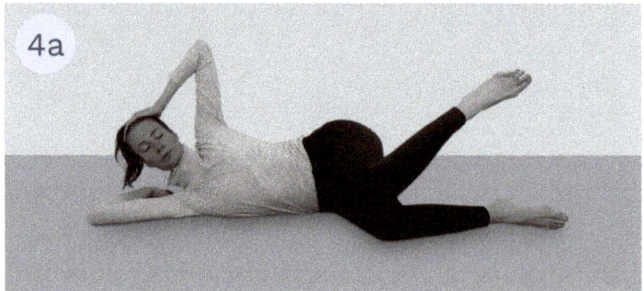

You may like to rest on your back before moving to the other side. Extend the legs and notice if one side feels longer/taller?

This movement is like an accordion opening and closing the side waist. Notice how as one side contracts the other side lengthens

Alternative arm positions

The straight arm position below can be an alternative when there are shoulder issues or having the arm bent over the head isn't comfortable. These variations can also help with stability and the idea of moving in a straight line, particularly if there is a tendency to round forwards or arch backwards when lifting.

3a] Straight arm: let the top arm rest long and straight along the topside of the body.

3a

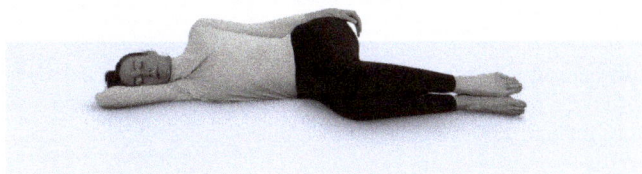

As you exhale and move into the pattern, reach away with the fingers – keeping that straight line as the arm lengthens away, contracting the waist. The head and neck lift in response

Releasing from the waist, returning everything to the starting position.

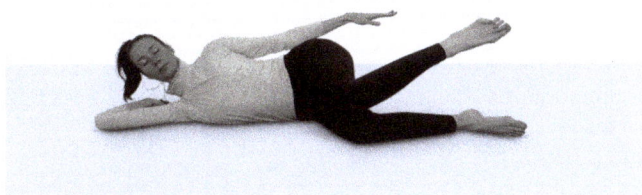

3b

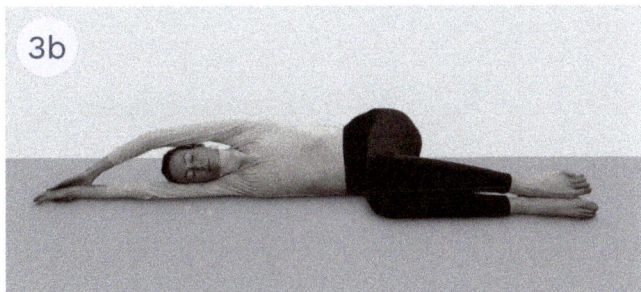

3b] Sweeping arm: here the arm position begins over the head. Inhaling to open and lengthen the sides of the body

Exhaling, sweeping the straight arm over as you move into the pattern.

The arm reaches away as the waist shortens, just as in the long arm movement above.

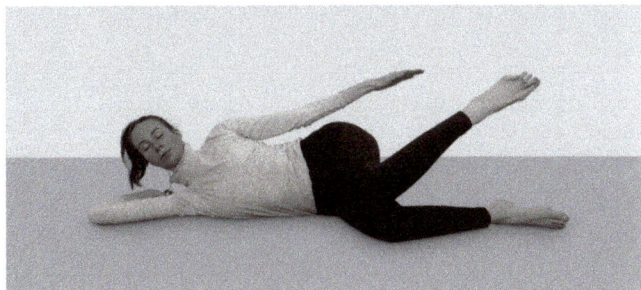

As you release from the centre of the waist you can either sweep the arm back over the head or just rest it down along the topside of the body.

Alternative leg position

An alternative leg position is to have the top leg straight. The long leg variation can combine well with the straight arm reaching away or the sweeping arm movement.

2a] Long leg variation: have the top leg straight.

The top leg extends long, the bottom leg is still bent for support and stability

Inhale length into the waist to set the movement up

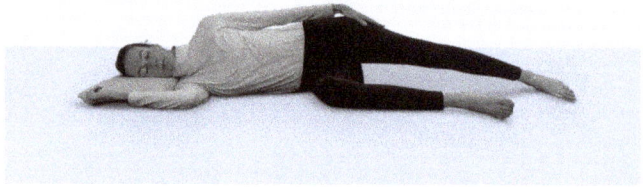

2a

Exhale, coordinate the waist and leg: the leg lifts in line and the side waist contracts and shortens to draw the hip and leg towards the armpit.

Release from the waist to lengthen and lower the leg back down.

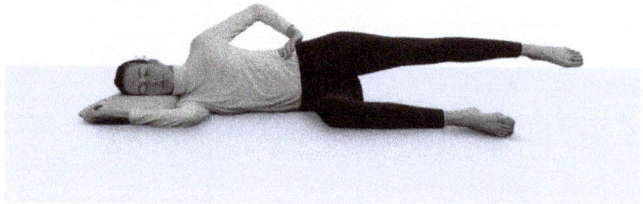

4b] Put together: The long leg variation can combine well with the straight arm reaching away (see 3.a) or the sweeping arm movement (see 3.b).

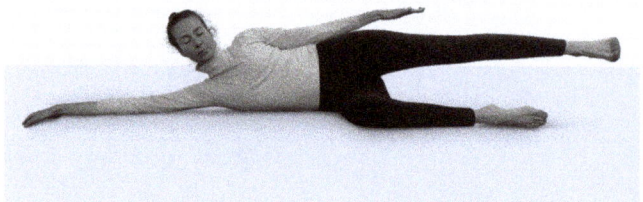

4b

PART FIVE

Spirals and integration

walking
patterns

Movement 10

Spirals (washrag)

This spiral-like movement is a helpful integrating movement that is useful to include towards the end of your practice.

This can also be a balancing movement when there are rotations, twists and pulls presenting in posture.

In clinical somatics you may see this called the 'washrag' as it is likened to the wringing of a wash cloth. As there are a lot of moving parts it can be helpful to build up to the full movement in stages.

1] Lie on your back, knees bent, feet flat to the floor.

Arms are along the floor, comfortably away from the body, beginning with **both palms facing up**.

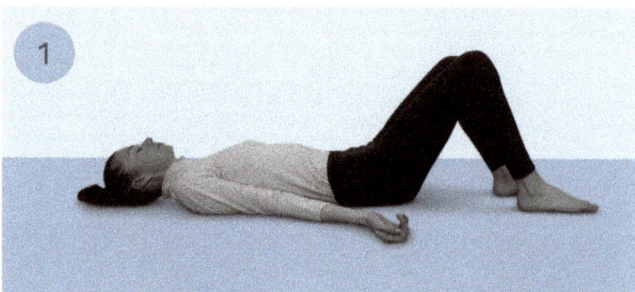

2] **Arm rotation:** roll one hand/arm/palm down, while the other stays up.

Then change both arms at the same time, alternating one up, one down. Connect the rotation up to the shoulders.

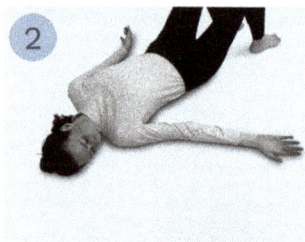

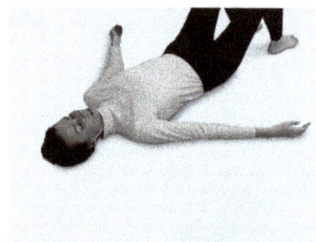

3] **Head:** Let the head roll with the movement, turning to face towards the side of the open arm/hand.

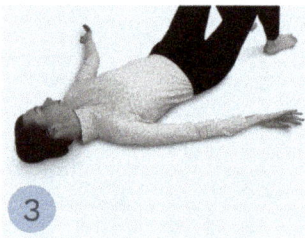

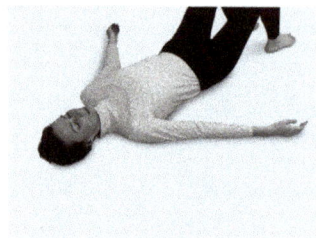

Let the movement rotate the whole arm, from the fingertips to the shoulder, like two rolling pins going in different directions. Make it a smooth alternating rotation of each arm, connecting up to the shoulders.

Movement 10 Spirals (washrag) continued

4] Add the knees: Pause in the movement, let the knees and pelvis flow over towards the side of the hand/arm facing down. The knees will move back and forth between left and right as you alternate with the arms.

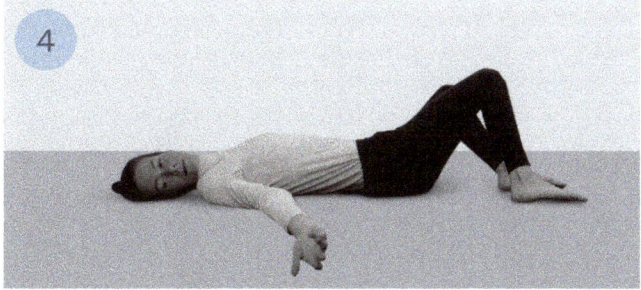

Remember this is a gentle lengthening through the waist (not a big stretch or arch).

Reverse the arms and legs flowing over to the other side, head moves too.

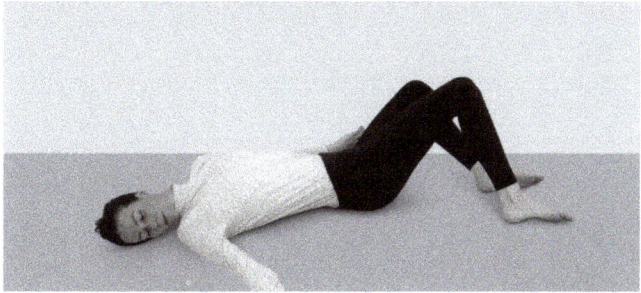

Explore this full movement: Knees towards the left, left arm/shoulder rotating in, right arm open, head looks to the right. Then reverse everything.

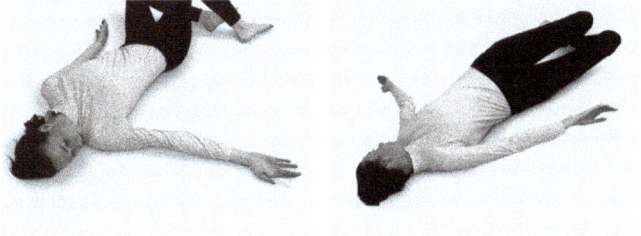

When first learning it can be helpful to remember the spiral pattern: **knees down** to the **hand down** side; **head** looks **up** to the **hand up** side. Then reverse everything

Movement 11

Walking Integration

These movements continue the theme of integration, specifically around patterns of walking and freeing up the pelvis, hips, lower back and waist to support this.

The two movements explore the different planes and ways that the pelvis moves in walking. It's like horizontal walking - we're exploring the movement patterns but by lying down.

It is important to move slowly and without going into any sensations of stretch or discomfort.

While these instructions use the knees and legs to initiate the movement, the important connection is the movement of the pelvis. You can place your hands on the hips as you explore these movement to notice the connection.

Part 1

1] Lie on your back, knees bent with **feet** planted **wide apart**

(if using a yoga mat then walk or step the feet out towards the edges).

Our focus side to start will be the right leg. The left leg will stay stationary.

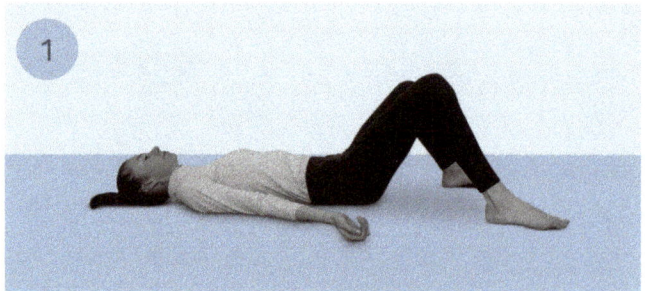

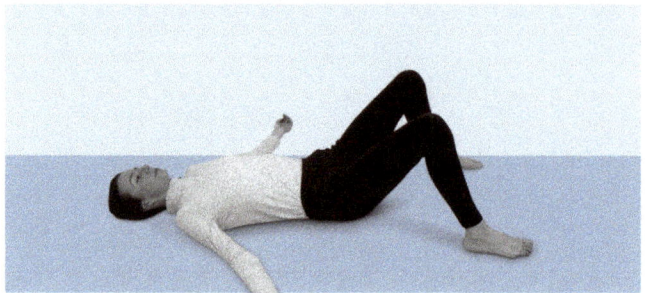

2] Let the **right knee** slowly **flow inwards** towards the midline and floor (rolling on the inside of your foot). The left leg stays stationary/upright.

Never force the knee down.

Return the right knee and hip to the starting position.

3] Explore this 3 times then repeat this for the left. *The right leg will stay stationary.*

4] You can then alternate moving left and then right. *As one leg returns up the other flows in.*

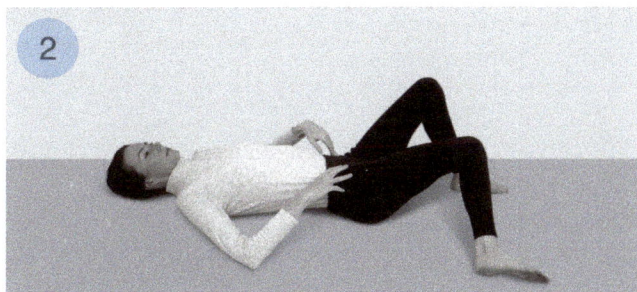

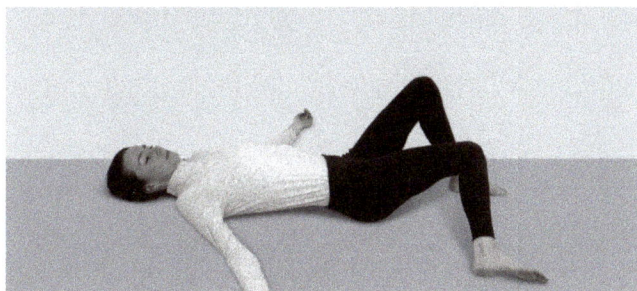

Notice how the muscles of the lower back, waist and front yield with the movement of the hip and leg. Feel the side-to-side shift of the pelvis as you move. You may even notice a connection up to the shoulders and that the head wants to roll to one side as you move the leg.

Somatic movement is mindful movement. Always work within your comfort range. Never force a movement or stretch to create a movement

Part 2

1] Lie on your back, knees bent, feet comfortably hip width apart.

(We've walked the feet back in after Part 1.)

Our focus side to start will be the right leg. The left leg will stay stationary.

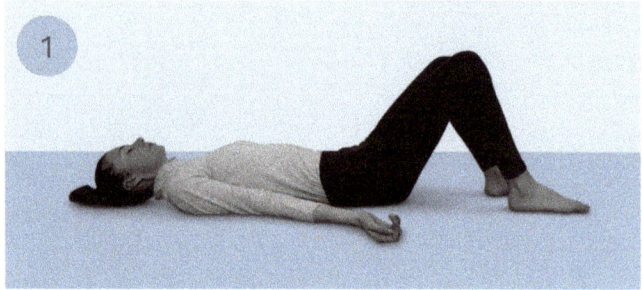

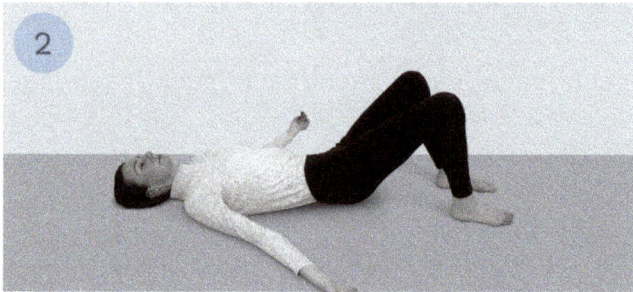

2] Press down through the right foot as you **send the right knee** and thigh **forwards** in space. The right hip will need to lift to allow this movement to happen. *It's like you are tapping an invisible wall in front with your knee. The right foot stays on the floor.*

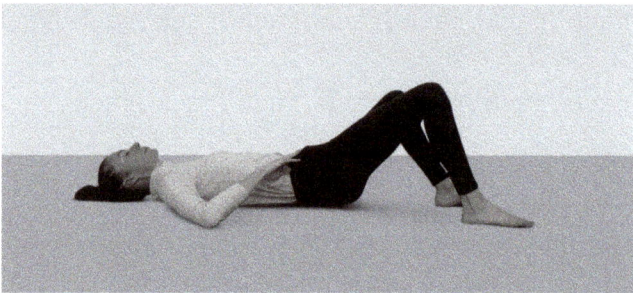

Lower the hip, buttock, pelvis back to the starting position (leg will follow).

Explore this movement a few times on the right. Sending the knee forwards. *Sense the yield of the waist and lower back.*

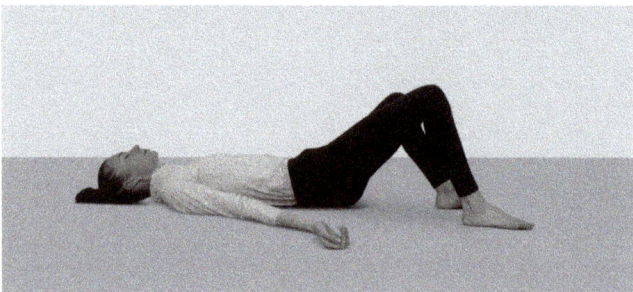

3] Then repeat this on the left, sending the left knee forwards. *The right leg will stay stationary.*

4] You can then alternate left and right. *Notice how the pelvis moves from side-to-side, coordinating and allowing this movement.*

Sensing
Body Scan (to end)

We end at the beginning, returning to the sensing body scan.

Noticing what has changed or is different, or may feel the same.

Not only does this give the brain and body time to integrate, it also lets us feel into a different possibility - one that you have the power to re-create.

1] Lie on your back with the arms and legs comfortably extended.

Allow your attention and awareness to turn inwards. Close the eyes if comfortable.

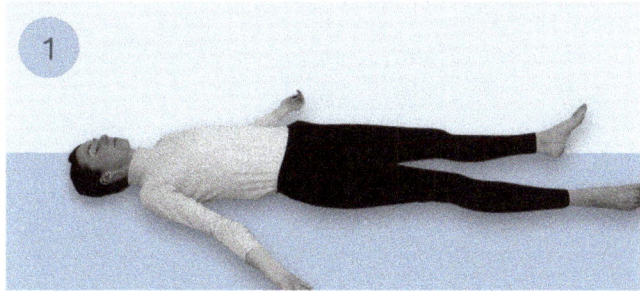

As you scan into the body you may notice

- The symmetry of the body, left and right.
- The upper and lower connections.
- The places of weight, contact and the curves and arches: around the ankles, behind the knees, the lower back, around the elbows and wrists.
- The shoulders left and right, and how the arms and hands are positioned.
- Checking in to the weight behind the head, and opening the eyes to see if the position of your gaze has changed. Notice how the neck feels.
- Gently and slowly roll the head left and then right, noticing the range and natural stop points either side.
- The constant companion of the breath, the place of the breath and if there is space for it to flow?
- How has this internal sense changed from the starting picture?
- How the mind, the whole interconnected you feels. Mind and body.
- As you prepare to move and return back into the world and life, do so slowly, bringing this somatic sense with you.
- Taking a walk afterwards can be further helpful integration, putting your movement practice into motion.

PART SIX

Next steps

Resources

Where to from here?

The end is just the beginning

Congratulations on learning and creating your smart muscles, smart brain movement toolkit.

It is not so much 'the end' here but the beginning. It is the beginning of cultivating your movement practice and deepening your somatic awareness.

The theory only works in practice.

The power in these foundational movements doesn't diminish once you've learnt them, the power is in using them. There is always more to learn and to explore, but having the core foundations to begin with, is key.

These become your movement toolkit, that you can continue to use, explore and take with you throughout life.

So you can keep doing the activities you love to do for as long as possible.

Revisit goals and photos

As you continue with your somatic movement practice revisit the earlier exercises. Review the goals you may have had and your earlier posture pictures.

Take new photos after a movement practice. Notice how your posture may have changed? Then how is it after a month, or three, six, a year from now? And importantly, how do you feel in yourself?

Small movements, done consistently becomes the change.

These movements offer an empowering tool for change. The smart muscles, smart brain way.

For more in the Smart Muscles Smart Brain series, including video and audio resources, visit: learnsomaticmovement.com

Wishing you mindful movement, with freedom and ease.

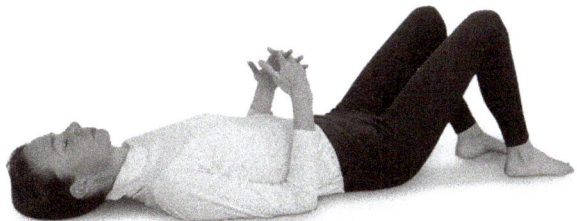

Sequence suggestions

Long practice

- Sensing Body Scan (start)
- M1 Finding Centre (arch/flatten)
- Include M2 Rebalancing if needed
- M3 Arch and Curl
- M4 Flower
- M5 Backlift 1
- M6 Backlift 2 (or M6 Variation)
- M7 Diagonal Arch and Curl
- M9 Sidebend (or M8 Gentle Waist)
- M10 Spiral Integration (washrag)
- M11 Walking Parts 1 & 2
- M1 Revisit briefly for symmetry
- Sensing Body Scan (end)

Medium practice

- Sensing Body Scan (start)
- M1 Finding Centre (arch/flatten)
- Include M2 Rebalancing if needed
- M3 Arch and Curl or M4 Flower
- M5 Backlift 1 or M6 Backlift 2
- M7 Diagonal Arch and Curl
- M9 Sidebend
- M10 Spirals (washrag)
- Sensing Body Scan (end)

Short practice

- Sensing Body Scan (start)
- M1 Finding Centre (arch/flatten)
- M3 Arch and Curl
- M8 Gentle Waist
- M10 Spirals (washrag)
- Sensing Body Scan (end)

Upper body focus

- Sensing Body Scan (start)
- M1 Finding Centre (arch/flatten)
- Include M2 Rebalancing if needed
- M8 Gentle Waist (with arms long)
- M3 Arch and Curl
- M4 Flower
- M6a Backlift Upper head/neck
- M7 Diagonal Arch and Curl
- M10 Spirals (washrag)
- Sensing Body Scan (end)

Lower body focus

- Sensing Body Scan (start)
- M1 Finding Centre (arch/flatten)
- Include M2 Rebalancing if needed
- M5 Backlift 1 (include legs)
- M7 Diagonal Arch and Curl
- M9 Sidebend
- M11 Walking Parts 1 & 2
- M10 Spirals (washrag)
- Sensing Body Scan (end)

Front focus

- Sensing Body Scan (start)
- M1 Finding Centre (arch/flatten)
- M2 Rebalancing Centre
- M3 Arch and Curl
- M4 Flower
- M7 Diagonal Arch and Curl
- M10 Spirals (washrag)
- Sensing Body Scan (end)

Back focus

- Sensing Body Scan (start)
- M1 Finding Centre (arch/flatten)
- M3 Arch and Curl
- M5 Backlift 1
- M6 Backlift 2 or Variations
- M7 Diagonal Arch and Curl
- M11 Walking Parts 1 & 2
- M10 Spirals (washrag)
- M1 Revisit briefly for symmetry
- Sensing Body Scan (end)

Sides focus

- Sensing Body Scan (start)
- M1 Finding Centre (arch/flatten)
- M2 Rebalancing Centre
- M8 Gentle Waist Movement
- M9 Sidebend
  + explore arm/leg variations
- M10 Spirals (washrag)
- Sensing Body Scan (end)

Diagonals and twists

- Sensing Body Scan (start)
- M1 Finding Centre (arch/flatten)
- M2 Rebalancing Centre
- M6 Backlift 2 (or variations)
- M7 Diagonal Arch and Curl
- M11 Walking Parts 1 & 2
- M10 Spirals (washrag)
- Sensing Body Scan (end)

The 'tech neck' offset

- Sensing Body Scan (start)
- M1 Finding Centre (arch/flatten)
- M8 Gentle Waist (with arms long)
- M4 Flower
- M5 Backlift 1
- M6a Backlift Upper head/neck
- M3 Arch and Curl
- M10 Spirals (washrag)
- Sensing Body Scan (end)

The deadline driven do-er

- Sensing Body Scan (start)
- M1 Finding Centre (arch/flatten)
- M3 Arch and Curl
- M5 Backlift 1
- M6 Backlift 2 or Variations
- M7 Diagonal Arch and Curl
- M10 Spirals (washrag)
- Sensing Body Scan (end)

Anxious times reset

- Sensing Body Scan (start)
- M1 Finding Centre (arch/flatten)
- M2 Rebalancing Centre
- M8 Gentle Waist Movement
- M3 Arch and Curl
- M4 Flower
- M7 Diagonal Arch and Curl
- M10 Spirals (washrag)
- Sensing Body Scan (end)

For more resources in the Smart Muscles Smart Brain program visit
learnsomaticmovement.com

Resources

Smart Muscles Smart Brain

Also available in the Smart Muscles Smart Brain series:

- Online Video Course
- Audiobook
- Ebook

For more resources or to find out about upcoming workshops and clinic dates visit: learnsomaticmovement.com

Somatic Movement Education Training

- Essential Somatics
  Martha Peterson
  essentialsomatics.com

Babies and Development

- Developmental Concept
  Karin Kalbantner-Wernicke and Dr. Thomas Wernicke
  developmentalconcept.com

Books

- Clear, J. (2018). *Atomic habits: tiny changes, remarkable results: an easy & proven way to build good habits & break bad ones.* New York: Avery, an Imprint of Penguin Random House.
- Doidge, N. (2007). *The Brain that Changes Itself: Stories of Personal Triumph from the Frontiers of Brain Science.* Melbourne: Scribe.
- Doidge, N. (2015). *The brain's way of healing : remarkable discoveries and recoveries from the frontiers of neuroplasticity.* New York, New York: Viking.
- Hanna, T. (2004). *Somatics : reawakening the mind's control of movement, flexibility, and health.* Cambridge, Ma: Da Capo Press.
- Levine, P.A. (1997). *Waking the tiger: Healing trauma: The innate capacity to transform overwhelming experiences.* Berkeley, Calif.: North Atlantic Books.
- Peterson, M. (2012). *Move Without Pain.* Union Square.
- van der Kolk, B. (2014). *The body keeps the score: brain, mind and body in the healing of trauma.* New York: Penguin Books.

About the author

Emily Harrison is a Certified Clinical Somatic Educator (CCSE) and somatic movement teacher.

Emily is also a practitioner of Shiatsu and Oriental Therapies, with specialist training in touch-based techniques to support early sensory-motor development, working with babies and children. She also draws on her background as a yoga and meditation teacher.

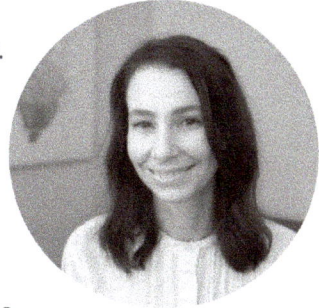

Based in Australia, Emily enjoys supporting people of all ages and life stages from newborns to the elderly.

Emily was drawn to somatic movement education having experienced first-hand the profound and empowering benefits that this system of neuromuscular education offers. She is the creator of the Smart Muscles Smart Brain program, weaving a developmental perspective alongside the foundational somatic movement exercises. This book is derived from her original video course resource, first launched online in 2022.

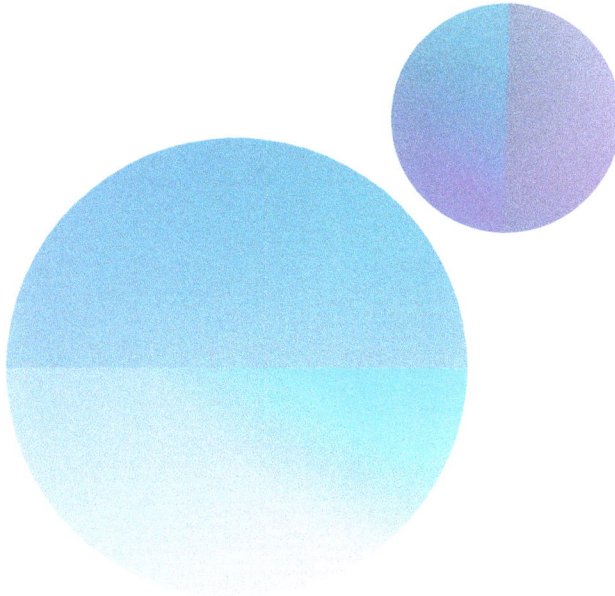